ASTHMA AND BRONCHITIS

Jan de Vries

Asthma and Bronchitis

By Appointment Only series

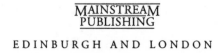

MAINSTREAM
PUBLISHING

EDINBURGH AND LONDON

First published in Great Britain in 1991 by
MAINSTREAM PUBLISHING COMPANY (EDINBURGH) LTD
7 Albany Street
Edinburgh EH1 3UG

This edition 2001

ISBN 1 84018 554 6

A catalogue record for this book is available from the British
Library

Typeset in Palatino
Printed and bound in Great Britain by Cox & Wyman Ltd

Contents

Foreword

WHAT CAN BE worse than a respiratory problem, being short of breath and always wheezing? I know, I have experienced it and, let's face it, if you don't breathe, you don't live! I was therefore pleased when Jan de Vries asked me to write the foreword to his latest book, on the subject of asthma and bronchitis, as I felt that this was the opportunity I had been waiting for to express my appreciation publicly for the help and guidance he has given me in my efforts to overcome a respiratory problem. He threw me a lifeline and, thank goodness, I had the sense to grab it with both hands.

Several years ago, following hospital tests, I was diagnosed as having bronchial asthma and was advised by conventional medical practitioners to use two different inhalers. Although I would have preferred to get to the bottom of the problem, at that time I was thankful for the help and relief provided by these inhalers, but I still couldn't help wondering what had brought on the asthma in the first place. Was it an allergy to certain items in my diet, a leftover from a cold, or perhaps something in the atmosphere? I felt there had to be a reason for it as I had always been blessed with good health. Anyway, I was obtaining a certain amount of relief from the inhalers but at the same time I was not happy about my constant use of them. Eventually I noticed the diminishing effect they were having and I began to have difficulty getting out to work in the mornings. One instance in particular stands out in my memory when I had to use my inhaler several times in order to make it.

This was when Jan de Vries took over. With patience and care he began to treat me with herbal and homoeopathic remedies, a little manipulation to help ease the breathing, and some advice on my diet. The latter is most important to respiratory sufferers, as I have proved to myself at times such as holidays and special celebrations like Christmas, when I have been tempted to stray from the "straight and narrow". The reader will no doubt find plenty of advice in this book which, if followed conscientiously, must surely give the desired results. I can only say that Jan de Vries was responsible for pointing me in the right direction, which eventually led me to completely conquer the asthma problem with which I had been plagued for years.

Now I am happy to say my quality of life has greatly improved. I go swimming several times a week, and I am back on the dance floor enjoying myself. I think I missed dancing more than anything during those years of misery, as I had been an ardent competitive dancer for many years and consequently became professional, but with the shortage of breath I was experiencing I eventually found it difficult to continue. Also, I can now go for long walks, even in the windy weather which is prevalent in the coastal town where I live. All this I can do again without any problem, thanks to Jan de Vries.

He is a most sincere and caring person and truly quite a remarkable practitioner. He has written many books now and I have read them all, but for me this book must surely be the greatest. Of course, it could be said that I am prejudiced!

I have therefore great pleasure in recommending this book to all who suffer breathing problems, as you must surely reap the benefit.

Isobel Fullarton
May 1991

1

Common Colds

I OFTEN HEAR FROM patients the expression "It started with a common cold". It is very likely that the common cold in question has been ignored and so has caused sometimes insurmountable problems. A common cold is often underestimated, yet it should never be neglected. People come to me complaining that they have had a cold for six weeks or longer, and a recurrent inflammatory condition or a wheeze is clear evidence that this cold has not cleared up and is ready to explode into something more difficult to treat.

Now, what really is a cold? *Merck's Manual* gives us a very clear definition: "an acute catarrhal infection of the respiratory tract usually with major involvement of its upper portions, and frequently involving the entire tract, referred to as an upper respiratory infection or *coryza* — the term used for acute nasal congestion."

There are many causes of a common cold and it is all

too often the case that it is the result of a virus. The nose, mouth and throat may become infected and inflamed, causing swelling, and sometimes such a viral infection leads to a secondary infection resulting in nasal discomfort, ranging from a watery to a thick yellow-greenish mucous discharge. In such cases common symptoms are a runny nose, sore throat, sneezing, watery eyes and headaches. When a person's immunity is low and the natural reserves are below par, for whichever reason, an ordinary common cold can result in a general debility such as a chronic infection, allergic disorders, vasomotor instability, injury to the mucous membranes and other such chronic conditions.

In many cases, however, the effects tend to be acute and can cause considerable discomfort, albeit for a relatively short period only. Sometimes the cold is accompanied by a fever, but with some sensible care the overall condition can soon be brought under control. On the whole the patient will be feeling much better within four to seven days.

However, in this book I intend to concentrate on the various conditions that could result from a common cold. I am well aware, having treated thousands of patients, that the after-effects often ascribed to a cold need not occur if sufficient care is taken in the first place. If common sense would only prevail I would be required to see fewer patients whose eventual chronic conditions can be traced back to a neglected common cold. Here we have the reason that I want to spend some time looking into the methods that can be employed to protect oneself when a cold strikes.

While I have been working on this book the weather has suddenly changed from being pleasantly mild to considerably chilly. In these circumstances the chance of infection caused by viruses is greatly increased. Unfortunately, many people forget to adapt their clothing to suit such weather by changing to woollen or cotton garments. Natural materials are always preferable to artificial fibres. People should particularly beware of draughts during a sudden change in temperature. In fact, draughts are often more damaging to the health than a sudden drop in the temperature itself. Always remember, however, that should the temperature change suddenly, there is no need to stay inside; by all means go out and enjoy the fresh air, but take care that you are suitably dressed for the elements. And again, beware of draughts.

It is also important to obtain sufficient rest, sleep and relaxation. When the body has become chilled, or when you have been out in the rain or snow, take a hot bath to get the circulation going again and so raise the body temperature. In this context I can advise a hot foot bath, especially if circumstances are such that it is not possible to totally immerse yourself in a hot bath.

Another very important factor when you are suffering from a cold is to try at all times to keep the nasal passages clear so that you can continue to breathe through the nose. Steam inhalation with the addition of some chamomile and Poho oil has a soothing effect on an inflamed respiratory tract and will aid the breathing.

As for dietary management, try and keep your diet very light. One rarely feels like eating heavy meals when feeling congested because of a cold. Make sure you drink plenty of fluids, especially fruit juices that are rich in vitamin C. Eat plenty of fresh vegetables and at such times I would also advise taking a vitamin C supplement.

Contrary to popular belief, it is unwise to clear the mucous membranes too often and too thoroughly. If you simply tilt your head backwards you will find it easier to breathe through the nose; this method is also less irritating. Should the cold linger, thereby obstructing

13

the nasal passages, try the age-old remedy of slicing an onion in half and placing both halves on a saucer by the bedside. This will bring speedy relief. Alternatively, some onion slices packed in a poultice around the throat will quickly ease the problem. You may prefer to use a nose douche prepared with a salt water solution, or to rub the chest with Poho ointment; both are excellent methods of overcoming a cold.

The first thing I would recommend in cases of a common cold is usually Dr Vogel's marvellous remedy Echinaforce. I could fill volumes on the remedial properties of Echinaforce and this remedy must be the one I have prescribed for more ailments than any other during nearly thirty years in medical practice. In cases of flu, cold, bronchitis, and many other types of infection, Echinaforce provides a tremendous boost to the immune system. At the University of Munich a lengthy study on Echinaforce has confirmed that it possesses properties that enhance the body's natural reserves. It seems that the polysaccharides it contains have a marked positive influence on immunity. It was also found that when viruses or micro-organisms try to spread through the body, Echinaforce has an hyaluronidase-slowing effect.

Let us remember that the white blood cells play a very important role in our immunity. Bacteria in the blood will be immediately attacked by the white blood cells and it may be astonishing to learn that a person with a body weight of 11–12 stones carries approximately 126,000,000 white blood cells in the bloodstream. These white blood cells act as defenders and with the right stimulating influence, i.e. a well-functioning immune system, they will rally into action and attack invaders. It also seems that the echinacea plant stimulates the production of natural interferon in the body. An added bonus is that Echinaforce has no side-effects whatsoever.

Over the years Professor H. Wagner, Head of the Institute of Pharmaceutical Biology at the University of Munich, has spent an enormous amount of time and energy researching the properties of echinacea. Although his research is still ongoing, he firmly believes that this wonderful remedy is of the greatest help in cases of infections — bacterial, viral and fungal.

My suggestion that Echinaforce should be taken immediately in cases of a common cold is based on my many years of experience. Moreover, the effects of this remedy can be enhanced when it is used in conjunction with the homoeopathic remedy *Kalium muriaticum* D6; this is especially true when the patient suffers from a blocked nose, a coated tongue, diminished hearing, an ear infection and a heavy mucus discharge. On the other hand if you are susceptible to infections, chronic sneezing, chapped lips, a dry mouth, or depressions, it would be advisable to use *Natrium muriaticum* D6.

When a cold refuses to disappear, people who are prone to such complaints would be advised to watch out for tiredness, high blood pressure, low temperature and depressive moods. Where children are concerned, it is especially important to check for swollen tonsils, breathing through the mouth, a chronic runny nose, excessive perspiration, a pale complexion and allergic reactions. Where these are noted dietary management should be given serious consideration. Wholefood products, including brown rice, plenty of fresh vegetables and fruit, a daily salad and the limited use of sugar and salt is important. Remember to eat slowly and be sure to include some cress, onions and garlic in the diet. People who are susceptible to the above symptoms would be wise to take a calcium supplement such as Urticalcin, which is an excellent combination of calcium silicum and one of the most popular calcium preparations as it

15

is quickly absorbed by the body. Also remember to take plenty of exercise in the fresh air and ensure ample rest at night.

When the lining of the mucous membrane is inflamed and irritated because of the extra mucus, action is needed to ease the resulting coughing. The inflamed mucous membranes must be soothed in an effort to stop their excess mucus production and to create an opportunity for the healing process to take effect. There are plenty of safe home remedies for this purpose, and especially in the case of a dry cough a cough mixture such as Drosinula syrup will be helpful. The flower on the cover of this book is one of the ingredients of this valuable remedy, which has proved especially effective in combating stubborn and deep coughs.

For children I often recommend Santasapina syrup, which is also an excellent remedy in cases of a dry cough. It is, of course, important when the coughing persists and no remedy appears to help that the advice of a doctor or qualified practitioner is sought. Irish moss and Iceland moss are also helpful, especially for diabetics who cannot take many standard cough mixtures.

A cold is a natural way of eliminating toxic waste material, which explains why herbal teas, such as hot elderflower tea or hot lemon and honey tea, are useful. Under such conditions it may also be wise to use such seasonings as cayenne, onions and garlic. I have been especially pleased to see how garlic has achieved wider recognition in recent years, as it is such a wonderful natural antibiotic and antiseptic. Whichever way it is taken, e.g. fresh, as capsules or tablets, or as a tincture, it will always give our health a little extra boost. The use of garlic goes back to ancient Egyptian times and it has become well known as a treatment for colds and flu. Whilst it is a completely safe and natural product without any side-effects, I would nevertheless confess to a slight hesitation at buying just any kind of garlic capsules. To my mind it is always best to use fresh garlic, as the substance called allicin that gives garlic its medical potency is produced when the enzyme allinase and the amino acid alinin, which are normally present in the garlic bulbs, are allowed to combine by crushing or heating. It is known that Chinese garlic, which is available from many chemists and health food stores, is generally of the highest quality. Back home in my younger days, when I helped out in a pharmacy, it was mostly the older generation who used to ask for fresh garlic capsules, as they were well aware of garlic's medicinal properties. For a long time garlic was almost taboo, as people disliked its characteristic taste and smell. Fortunately, nowadays there are some excellent garlic capsules and tablets on the market, in which the taste and odour has been largely eliminated.

In the case of acute colds characterised by a desperately runny nose, garlic and onions are often of great help. And I have been told that in the Highlands of Scotland an old-fashioned remedy of a plate of hot porridge with some onions and garlic is still being used for common colds. The older generation of farmers in Switzerland had their own cold cure: after harvesting the oats they used to make an infusion of the straw, which was found to be highly effective for treating cases of catarrh, coughs and feverish conditions.

Another popular remedy in medical folklore was horseradish syrup and especially in cases of persistent colds and catarrh it was customary to prepare a horseradish syrup with added sugar and honey. All the ingredients were mixed well and pressed through a sieve before being cooked with a little water and sugar to produce a syrup. This syrup will greatly relieve the symptoms of colds and chills. It is particularly important not to ignore catarrhal conditions and the old naturopathic methods of treatment are obviously still very effective.

The word catarrh has its roots in the Greek language; it is based on the two words *kata* (down) and *rhein* (to flow) and the combination of these two words is an apt description of the symptoms. A persistent and excessive flow of mucus can be the first indication of a chronic condition and the body should be stimulated to heal itself in order to get rid of unnecessary catarrhal problems. The lungs are understandably one of the body's most vulnerable organs and it is often the case that a long-term congestion has resulted from an apparently ordinary common cold. If the early signs that a cold is developing into a chronic catarrhal condition are heeded, further complications can be avoided. However, it never does any good to suppress a cold as eventually this could exacerbate the problem. Instead, allow the cold to run its course and alleviate the symptoms with some of the natural remedies mentioned earlier.

In 1946 the Medical Research Council established a Common Cold Research Centre in Salisbury, where for ten-day periods members of the public, who had volunteered to take part in the research programme, were kept in isolation from the outside world. The results were disappointing insofar that only very few viruses could be isolated and the only meaningful results from these tests were that viruses can only flourish under certain conditions. For this reason we should do our best to ensure that the immune system remains as healthy as possible, and believe me when I say that no worthwhile investment in one's health can ever be too expensive!

In cases of an infectious illness it is dangerous to consider the invisible virus as an enemy that can be destroyed by a drug, as is so often the case in conventional medicine. Samuel Hahnemann, the founder of homoeopathy, had the vision to recognise the danger of destroying one thing with another, for when we set out to destroy harmful bacteria, it is more than likely that beneficial bacteria will be killed off in the process.

A naturopathic practitioner will always look for the cause of the symptoms and by treating the cause may well cure the symptoms. Catarrhal conditions certainly can result from a common cold and the same is often true of other toxic conditions. The body is quite miraculous. If we help it positively in one way or another, the most simple remedies can often give the body the extra help that is needed to cure itself. The body does not like to be sick, it wants to be healthy, but it needs to be treated correctly.

The first step should be to look at our daily food intake, and try to eliminate the foods which aggravate the mucous membranes and form catarrh. A mucus-reducing diet is of great importance. It is well known that faulty nutrition aggravates catarrhal conditions. Avoid dairy products as much as possible and, if necessary, drink goat's milk or soya milk instead. Also avoid white sugar and white flour, especially white-flour products which contain a relatively high proportion of starch and have a reduced fibre content.

Another aspect that should be taken into account with colds and catarrhal conditions is the blood circulation. Our forebears were not so daft when they said that cold and frosty weather would kill off germs. There is probably a lot of wisdom in getting out into the fresh air, especially on a clear, sunny and frosty day. Not only does this provide our quota of oxygen, but the breathing and pumping of oxygen through the bloodstream will remove some of the waste material.

19

Lack of physical exercise can be another factor contributing to catarrh. I often wonder when I consider the increase in bronchial and asthmatic problems whether it might partly be due to lack of exercise, as the symptoms often go hand in hand with poor circulation. We often see that the lymphatics, which have an important function in maintaining good health, will work more effectively when circulation can take place unhindered. Good circulation can be seen as a muscular pump. Therefore exercises are important and none more so than breathing exercises. Some of the water treatments described in my book *Water — Healer or Poison?* will usually have a beneficial effect. A few days' fasting cannot do any harm either. Stay in bed and fast sensibly and this will serve as a very simple cleansing programme; instead of solid food, restrict yourself to liquids, i.e. water or fruit juices. During a fast, practise breathing exercises, possibly including some of the old-fashioned Kneipp treatments. In Chapter 12 I will outline some additional exercises which are useful for these conditions.

When dealing with catarrh and other cold-related problems it is often a question of common sense; nevertheless, it cannot be overstated that ignoring such symptoms will never do. Over the years I have seen so many problems that have been caused by people ignoring the early warning signs. It is therefore essential that we use our common sense to prevent any further development of such conditions. By considering a natural approach to the problem and encouraging it to work its way out of the system, rather than suppressing it, we can benefit. There is many a lesson we can learn from previous generations who lived so much closer to nature and followed their instincts. The application of mustard plasters or flax seed poultices were often used successfully to relieve quite severe chest discomforts.

During my pharmaceutical training I heard a story about a pharmacist who in 1890, in his drugstore in North Carolina, produced a now very well-known common cold ointment called Vick's Vapour Rub. It was during the American Civil War when the pharmacist, Lunsford Richardson, developed Vick's Vapour Rub, in which he used Japanese menthol, for his own five-year-old son. It seems astounding that by 1907, after this pharmacist had commercially developed his vapour rub, it was already being used all over the world. For nearly a century this product has been used by millions of people — and quite rightly so. It is also helpful to rub the chest with products such as Poho ointment, and other peppermint and menthol ointments. We can often benefit greatly from such simple remedies at times when our immune system is under attack.

Please take heed, however, that when using such vapour rubs on the chest, one should always take extreme care to stay out of draughts. Rub it gently into the skin of the chest and then cover the area with a woollen garment to keep it warm. Prevention is better than cure, so take proper action when caught out by an ordinary common cold and in this way you may be able to prevent some of the other conditions that I deal with later in this book. Remember how much help can be found in nature and it will point us in the right direction for treating some of these more serious conditions.

2

Bronchitis

MORE AND MORE I hear patients claim that their bronchial problems are a result of the weather. However, we must realise that this is usually used as an excuse, as it is more likely that acute or chronic bronchitis is the result of poor dietary management, smoking or other inflammations affecting the bronchial tubes that may be caused by infections or chemical influences.

Bronchitis is one of the most prevalent major lung diseases nowadays. Knowing this fact, the question must arise as to why this should be the case. The lungs are two sponge-like respiratory organs in the chest, whose function is to supply oxygen to and remove carbon dioxide from the blood. Of course, there are several reasons why our lungs can become overloaded. In the lifespan of an average person these sponge-like organs in the chest are filled with air approximately 500 million times. Special agents help these vital organs in this life-supporting job.

The tender tissue in the lungs is warmed and moisturised and contains a special enzyme which kills the air-borne bacteria. Glandular action is geared to aiding the air canals to function correctly and effectively. However, through poor breathing or smoking, along with other detrimental influences, we abuse these very tender bronchi to the extent that the approximately 750 million lung blisters become over-extended. It is then that problems such as asthma, bronchitis or emphysema can easily arise.

Sometimes, mainly in the case of acute bronchitis, a reaction occurs in the upper respiratory function which may be the result of a common cold, an infection of the nasal pharynx or the trachea-bronchial tree, or may be caused by a flu virus. This is the reason that bronchitis is more prevalent in winter than in summer and special care should always be taken to ensure that this condition does not develop into pneumonia. Recurring attacks of sinusitis, bronchiectasis, or allergy factors may also lead to an acute attack of bronchitis. An inflammation that may initially be caused by an allergic reaction to mite, dust, tobacco or some other substance may subsequently develop into tracheitis or bronchitis. Fortunately, acute bronchitis can be easily diagnosed, which is important because it can soon develop into chronic bronchitis, which is a long-standing condition of the trachea-bronchial tree characterised by chronic inflammation and fybrotic inflammation in the mucous membranes and deeper bronchial structures and is usually related to emphysema or other chronic conditions. In the latter conditions we usually find that the bronchi thicken and that the mucous glands and muscular layers become inflamed. This is often followed by obstruction of the ear passages and sometimes breathing difficulties. Swollen mucous membranes, which can lead to spasms of the bronchial muscles, tend to obstruct the ear passages and produce an obstructive ventilatory insufficiency. Any imbalance in the body chemistry, especially with chronic bronchitis, is often severe. Chest expansion and the individual's vital capacity are diminished, which can ultimately lead to emphysema. Once bronchitis has become chronic, it is difficult to cure, unless the patient undergoes proper treatment to control not only the cough, but also the production of mucus.

It is therefore good to know that phytotherapy and homoeopathic remedies combined with sensible dietary measures can bring great relief when suffering from such conditions. For either acute or chronic bronchitis it is advisable to use Usneasan. If preferred, this remedy is also available in the form of tablets which can be sucked in the same way as a cough sweet.

It is most important to pay due attention to one's dietary management and, in particular, to avoid all dairy products. Adopt a well-balanced diet rich in vitamins A and C, while also making good use of the ingredients I have already mentioned such as honey, onions and garlic. A multivitamin preparation which also contains the minerals selenium and zinc will be of help, as will royal jelly, pollen and propolis. Together with some extra vitamins A and C, this will provide a good basis for treating bronchitis.

It is also important that smokers, who inhale millions of little nicotine particles, are fully aware how negative an influence this habit is for people who are inclined to suffer from either acute or chronic bronchitis. It may be frightening to realise that if a person smokes twenty cigarettes a day, by the age of fifty this will have amounted to nearly 220,000 cigarettes.

It is also often the case that people who are more than usually susceptible to bacteria and viruses are prone to bronchitis. Oddly, it appears that this is more common in men than in women, but it is a growing problem universally. When the white blood cells become overloaded, a chronic bronchitis attack can lead to a problem that resembles a severe attack of flu and certainly to a disturbance in the breathing function, resulting in a persistent cough. Chronic bronchitis is the cause of excessive mucus production and coughing, especially during the night, which will make the patient restless and nervous, further aggravating the problem.

If this condition is allowed to deteriorate, the blood will be unable to absorb sufficient oxygen, leading to further coughing and breathing difficulties. An airless, smoky atmosphere can be extremely damaging to bronchitis patients and may even lead to bronchiectasis and emphysema. I come across this frequently in the case of farmers, who are often required to work under damp conditions; the subsequent development of bronchitis that occurs sometimes leaves them severely handicapped.

This condition can be kept in check to a large extent by restricting oneself to a wholefood diet from which all dairy produce is banned. Milk and cheese are among the most detrimental foods in the diet of a bronchitis sufferer. Although cow's milk is rich in calcium, it is badly lacking in magnesium and iron. Another problem is that milk contains casein. It is very hard for the human body to assimilate milk and when a baby is weaned from its mother's milk we often recognise the first signs of allergies, such as infantile eczema or catarrhal conditions which stem from enzymatic changes and the inability to digest dairy products, especially because of the casein factor. This, of course, is because of the pasteurisation, which is unavoidable. It is often even more difficult to properly digest evaporated milk, long-life milk and skimmed powdered milk, because the heat treatment

25

these products are subjected to results in lack of digestive enzymes. Peptides are a compound formed from two or more amino acids by the linkage of amino groups of some of the acids or by hydrolysis of proteins, and where the digestive enzymes are lacking these peptides cannot be properly absorbed. In these circumstances the immune system deals with the peptides as a foreign protein, with the result, especially in young children, that the body begins to build up an immunity to these proteins and we have the start of allergic conditions. Poor digestion often leads to poor absorption, which in turn leads to other problems.

We should now see why dietary management is so important for the control of both acute and chronic bronchitis and why it is essential to follow a regular system of rebuilding one's health. Disease of the lungs and the bronchial tubes may be treated following the naturopathic approach, which enables us to deal with the real underlying cause of the trouble. Also, I should point out how important it is to pay attention to the kidneys because in cases of chronic bronchitis in particular, the kidneys will not be functioning at their full capacity. To compensate for this it would be wise to drink herbal tea. Garlic capsules, peppermint oil, Obbekjaer's peppermint powder or pills are all useful for this purpose too. Biochemical remedies such as *Ferr. phos.* will also help to reduce the temperature; this is often taken in combination with *Kali. mur.* or *Nat. mur.*

Although bronchitis is rarely fatal, it can easily develop into a permanent and recurring affliction if the patient's general health is below par. Prevention is better than cure and therefore when acute infections are repeatedly experienced it is important that some preventative care is taken. When living in a damp climate it is helpful to take the occasional holiday in a mild and sunny climate to minimise the risk of contracting irritating conditions and, of course, remember to use the relevant remedies.

I remember an elderly farmer who was totally averse to any dietary treatment or remedies, but his bronchial condition finally became so debilitating that he was forced to seek help. In the event he wrote to me after visiting the clinic:

"Thank you for the very effective treatment I received for my bronchitis. I have been dogged by this complaint for quite a few years, but now I am feeling so much better. The treatment you prescribed has done me the world of good and I now feel better than I have felt for years. Thank you very much indeed."

Such letters are encouraging for the practitioner, because it is not always easy when people look at me with an expression of incredulity on their faces when I advise them to use some of the simple remedies I have mentioned earlier, or when I suggest that they would do well to change their dietary habits. Of course I understand that it is not always the most popular solution when a patient is told that his or her diet may have to be revised, because most people are in a hurry to improve their condition and feel that even if dietary measures were to be effective, the process would take too long.

Sometimes it is useful to eliminate just one food item at a time from the diet. In cases of bronchitis the first of these items should be dairy products. You do get used to it, and many of these products can be replaced by goat's milk or soya milk products. When you begin to feel the effects of such dietary changes you will pluck up the courage to experiment further. There is no sense in becoming fanatical about it, but try to relate to the body that you want to help and, above all, approach it in a sensible manner. The body will be thankful for any help that is offered and I have heard from countless patients that they feel so much better afterwards. With that in mind I will conclude this chapter with a recommended diet, which I have worked out over the years according to the feedback I have received from asthma and bronchitis patients.

Diet for asthma and bronchitis patients

Breakfast:
Grapes, grapefruit or stewed apple with prunes.
Muesli, porridge with molasses or honey and soya milk.
Cornflakes; All-Bran or raw oats with soya milk; molasses
   and water; watery apple juice or prune juice.
Brown rice and/or cooked barley with soya sauce.
Two slices of rye crispbread.

Lunch:
A salad containing any raw vegetable except tomatoes.
   Any cabbage-based salad is very good.
Onions, garlic and sprouts.
Blended vegetable soup made with Plantaforce.
Two slices of rye crispbread or one slice of pumper-
   nickel.
Jacket potato, brown rice, cooked millet or a mixture of
   cooked millet, potato and/or barley.

Supper:
Lamb — no more than twice a week.
Beef — only once a week.
Game — no more than twice a week.
Non-oily sea fish — no more than twice a week.
Eggs — a maximum of two per week and in severe cases
   eggs should be eliminated completely.
Liver or kidneys — only once a fortnight.

Pulses combined from soya, aduki, haricot and kidney beans, lentils or chickpeas — at least twice a week.

Tofu.

Cooked fresh vegetables, sea vegetables and bean sprouts.

Potatoes and/or whole grains, i.e. rice, millet, millet and potato, or barley.

At least one day a week eat meals consisting of fruit, vegetables and whole grains only.

Any fruit except oranges, but only a limited quantity of bananas.

Any puddings that do not contain cow's milk or wheat flour.

Beverages:

China, Earl Grey or 100% Herbal Health tea without milk or sugar.

Herb teas, especially rose hip and peppermint with a sprinkling of hops. Sage and thyme tea (one cup per day).

A cup of hot, boiled water sipped first thing every morning.

Spring water, vegetable and fruit juices (unsweetened and diluted). Apple juice and beetroot juice are especially beneficial.

Dressings, oils and condiments:

Dress salads with Molkosan, olive oil and lemon juice or cider vinegar. Garlic in the dressing is beneficial.

For cooking, use sunflower, soya or olive oil.

Herbs, spices, Herbamare.

Honey, molasses or brown sugar may be used in moderation.

Dietary supplements:

One tablet of Immuno-strength (Nature's Best) twice daily.

1,000 mg vitamin C.
500 IU vitamin E.
Four kelp tablets daily.

Foods to avoid:
Cow's milk and all related products, i.e. cheese, skimmed milk, evaporated and long-life milk, butter and cream, except natural yoghurt. Use goat's yoghurt where possible. Pork and related products, i.e. bacon, ham, and sausages. Tomatoes, malt vinegar, red wine, white sugar, chocolate, and common salt. Reduce the intake of bread or cooked wheat-flour products, coffee, and smoked, pickled or convenience foods.

Finally, I would add that for bronchitis patients it is very important that in conjunction with the diet some vitamin, mineral and trace element supplements are used, and by that I mean a full spectrum of supplements. For this purpose I would recommend Health Insurance Plus from the Nature's Best range. Also from the same range I can heartily recommend a new addition to their product range called Ester-C; this unique form of vitamin C has been granted an American patent and has been shown in tests to be three times more bioavailable than ordinary vitamin C. Ester-C enters the blood in half the time of ordinary ascorbic acid. Twice as much of it gets to the blood, where it can circulate to all the tissues of the body — and it stays in the body twice as long. The body tissues appear to take up four times more Ester-C than ascorbic acid and "waste" only a third as much. Volunteers who took the new Ester-C reported fewer stomach upsets, which occasionally occur when taking large amounts of vitamin C. Ester-C also seems to have removed another concern, in that it appears less likely to contribute to the formation of the chemicals known as oxalates which, when found in urine, are associated with kidney stones. I consider this a very exciting new discovery and a genuine breakthrough in the supply of what may be our most important single nutrient. After talking to my friend Jeffrey Bland, who has been testing this product for some time, I have learned that this product is of tremendous value for all asthma and bronchitis cases.

3

Bronchiectasis

BRONCHIECTASIS IS A chronic congenital disease characterised by cystic dilation of the bronchial mucosa. The term bronchiectasis indicates an infection or obstruction and these infections may be secondary to pneumonia, silicosis, emphysema or other infectious conditions. Once the bronchial mucosa has become inflamed or ulcerated there may be blood in the sputum as a result of small haemorrhages and abscesses. A person affected by this condition is often subject to recurrent attacks and the more uptight and tense the patient becomes at the thought of an oncoming attack, the harder it is for him or her to cope with it. Sputum in every form is evident; sometimes it is frothy, greenish and thick and sometimes it is very difficult to bring up as the congestion is such that it really requires treatment. Breathing is often difficult and severe coughing bouts can sometimes lead to exhaustion as the body tenses itself for every attack. Drainage can be very helpful, but this will have to be repeated from time to time. Sometimes oxygen or compressed air will have to be used, and antispasmodics will also be called for to ease the condition in severe cases.

The bronchiectasis patient is very sensitive to infectious conditions and must therefore take care as any infection will aggravate the problem. I have already mentioned a number of breathing exercises such as the Hara breathing technique, which is described in detail in Chapter 12, and bronchiectasis patients would be well advised to familiarise themselves with it. The importance of correct breathing will become evident if we consider the fact that each individual inhales and exhales about 500 million times during an average life span. This action is absolutely vital to our existence as the oxygen is transported by our bloodstream to each and every cell in the body.

Every minute we inhale and exhale between ten and sixteen times and in so doing we transport approximately sixteen pints of air, which means that each day we breathe in about 20,000 pints of air. So, in this life process the breathing activity has to be as efficient as possible. It is essential that oxygen is inhaled in the first place before the body can do anything with it. Oxygen, which is soluble in water, will travel through the cell wall to be changed into CO_2. Air reaches the lungs via the nose and mouth. In the nose there is a very rich membrane that filters the air and keeps it moist so that dust can be controlled. Via the nose, the air reaches the throat and passes down the trachea. The trachea is a cylindrical drain, 12 cm long and 2 cm in diameter; the wall of the trachea contains cartilage and is very strong. The trachea then separates into two bronchi, respectively the bronchioli and the respitory of the breathing bronchioli. These support the lungs to do their job of breathing properly. Remember that these roads come to an end in many millions of lung blisters, where a change is effected and from where the pulmonary artery transports the oxygen through the bloodstream by way of the heart.

The efficient function of the heart and lungs ensures the vitally important oxygen supply to every blood cell. This process is interactive and it is therefore essential that all stages of the process run smoothly. The muscles and organs participating in this process require simple and gentle exercise so that they all can function and perform well. Breathing in and out very gently is essential for each and every person and never more so than for the bronchiectasis patient. Sometimes if he or she feels very tired it is helpful to bend over, place the head between the arms and rest it on a table, keeping the arms wrapped loosely around the head. Breathe gently, in through the nose, all the way deep down into the stomach and out again through the mouth. This procedure could hardly be simpler and yet it will bring great relief.

The carbon dioxide content of the blood must constantly be kept at the correct level for the body to function efficiently. Back in 1928 scientists discovered what is now called the pneumotaxic centre, which looks after the rhythmic activity of the breathing process. Nerve impulses originate in the pneumotaxic centre, which control the constant rhythm of inhalation and exhalation. So, all together, we are looking at a system which is designed to work at maximum efficiency, if possible without any coughing spells — and our body does it all for us. Unless there is a disorder we never give this matter a second thought.

I have been in practice in Scotland for more than twenty years, and during that time I have been approached for help by many bronchiectasis patients, most of them coming from the many small mining communities. I have seen numerous patients who have come to me over the years with bronchiectasis or emphysema, all at various stages of developing a chronic bronchial condition. One can only conclude that the inhalation of materials which irritate the air channels is one of the most likely causes, aggravated sometimes by tiredness, poor nutrition, a low level of immunity, viral infection and air pollution. The first signs a bronchiectasis patient will note are often a dry cough, a gradual constriction of the air canals and feeling of tightness in the chest.

I was born and raised in a Dutch town where the main employers were involved in the tobacco industry. Like many others, my father, before he changed his lifestyle, worked in the tobacco industry. I will never forget how sorry I felt, as a youngster, for our coughing and asthmatic friends and acquaintances and for those who suffered from more serious conditions such as tuberculosis, pneumonia and emphysema. It is sad to see that some of these conditions are becoming more familiar again nowadays, not because of poor working conditions, but because of poor quality food and a lowering of the effectiveness of the immune system as a result of atmospheric influences that irritate and deplete our reserves. If a bronchiectasis patient smokes I cannot stress enough that he or she should immediately give up that addictive habit and also that care is taken to avoid smoky surroundings. Be wary of sudden temperature changes also, either moving from the cold to the warmth, or vice versa. If possible, take your holidays in the mountains to enjoy the clean air or, failing that, choose to spend your holidays in warm and dry climates.

Aromatherapy is an appropriate form of therapy for bronchiectasis patients, especially with the oils of lemon, eucalyptus, hyssop, myrrh, oregano, sandal-wood, peppermint, thyme and salvia. People suffering from this condition should also drink plenty of fluids, as well as using honey, garlic and vitamins A and C. Again, please refrain from all dairy products. Introduce plenty of fresh fruit and vegetables into the diet and as far as minerals are concerned, the main ones to remember are selenium and zinc. Beta carotene, which is important for bronchiectasis patients, can be obtained from carrots and also in tablet form. The anti-oxidant supplied by vitamin A will help with all lung diseases, including lung cancer. It is important for such patients to eat plenty of dark vegetables and fruits, such as carrots, spinach, broccoli, apricots, endive, curly kale, potatoes, lettuce, beetroot and turnips; these all have properties that help to stimulate the immune system. Cod liver oil will often be of help too.

Although bronchiectasis is often treated by drugs, do not forget that effective alternative treatments are available. These patients often have a tendency to be depressed or downhearted and frequently experience panic attacks. Some especially helpful remedies can be found in homoeopathy and phytotherapy, for example, *Bryonia, Kali sulph., Kali. iod.* or Guajacum. The old-fashioned remedy horseradish syrup will prove helpful, as will extra calcium and Immunoforce (Formula IMN), the immunity- boosting formula from the Bioforce range, together with Petaforce or Brochosan. Rubbing the chest with some Poho oil often brings relief to the bronchiectic patient. Finally, a course of soft tissue manipulation or acupuncture treatment sometimes helps to relieve this persistent affliction.

4

Emphysema

EMPHYSEMA IS A localised condition that has developed into an acute or chronic loss of elasticity and overdistension of the pulmonary alveoli. These become distorted and can sometimes rupture or allow air to enter into the tissues. There are many kinds of emphysema, the most common being the peribronchial or bronchioli obstruction, which is mainly associated with chronic bronchitis or asthma.

In cases of emphysema the lungs are somewhat dry and prone to collapse, with subsequent damage to the thorax. In many cases there are adhesions and air sacs and often the bronchi are subject to chronic infection and loss of elasticity because the alveoli walls are defective. The vascular problems and impaired circulation experienced by many emphysema patients can also contribute to an inadequate supply and transportation of oxygen.

Many emphysema patients become easily fatigued and suffer from insomnia and lack of appetite. Their energy reserves are likely to be below par and therefore they can be quickly debilitated by the chronic coughing and shortage of breath. Such patients may well suffer from bronchiectasis, with the complication of severe and recurrent bouts of coughing. If a case of emphysema has become chronic, great care should be taken to watch out for signs of infection or cardiac problems. In cases of younger people who have been diagnosed as having emphysema the cause is often postural. Once the posture of these patients has been examined to identify the cause of any blockages, simple exercises can be suggested to overcome this condition. Regular swimming is highly recommended for such youngsters and they will soon notice an improvement if they follow this advice. Tension causes the greatest discomfort to all emphysema patients and therefore stress or nervous tension should be avoided at all costs.

On a recent flight to the United States I was sitting next to a person whom I immediately recognised as suffering from emphysema. The gentleman concerned, I could observe, had a rather thin skin and I could also hear that his breathing was laboured. He was extremely nervous, so I chatted away to him in an effort to distract him. Some time later I enquired if he suffered from an asthmatic condition. When this was confirmed I asked if I could hazard a guess and suggested that he was plagued by emphysema symptoms. He wondered how I was able to tell just by looking at him and said that no one had ever remarked upon it except occasionally to notice his shortness of breath. I informed him that I could also see that he was undergoing steroid treatment because of the thinning of his skin and added that most likely he was suffering from a thinning of the bones.

I have often found with asthmatic or bronchiectic patients, and especially with those suffering from emphysema, that the situation has become so difficult that the practitioner has had no other choice than to prescribe steroids. The effects of this form of treatment become clearly noticeable by the thinning of the skin and bones. During my chat with my fellow traveller I volunteered some dietary advice and I also enquired whether he took any calcium supplements. He declared that this had never been suggested to him before. I also gave him some advice regarding relaxation exercises that he could practise when an attack came on, instead of hurriedly searching for his inhaler, or for yet another Prednisilone tablet, or for that matter any kind of medication that people use to try to stop the onset of a sudden attack.

I have often seen that a few simple adjustments to the diet combined with natural or homoeopathic medication can do much to help the condition. Moreover, people undergoing long-term steroid treatment should be warned of the possible side-effect known as osteoporosis. This condition of demineralisation of the bones, with an increaing tendency towards porosity, is closely associated with a shortage of calcium and vitamin D, too little physical movement, poor absorption of vitamins and minerals, an excess of phosphorous, hormonal imbalances, an excess intake of meat, and stress. It can result in weakened and painful bones, back problems and deformities of the bone structure. Therefore it is especially recommended that patients undergoing long-term steroid treatment follow a well-balanced diet rich in minerals such as calcium, magnesium and silicea. They should take care to eat plenty of yoghurt, vegetables (both raw and cooked), sesame and/or sunflower seeds. Products containing white sugar and white flour should be kept to a minimum, as should tinned products. It is also advisable to eliminate meat from the diet; if you feel you cannot do this, then it should be eaten in small amounts only. It is important to take plenty of vitamins A, B_{12}, C, D and E, and from the mineral range calcium, dolomite, copper, iron, magnesium, silicea and fluoride. Herbal drinks containing alfalfa, nettle and comfrey are beneficial. Also, when the symptoms of osteoporosis become apparent, it is helpful to use Symphytum and Urticalcin, both of which are products from the Bioforce range.

I have already mentioned the importance of relaxation for emphysema patients and this reminds me of an elderly shepherd who used to attend my clinic. For many years he had coped with his emphysema problems better than most. The secret of his success was mainly that he had a relaxing job and spent most of his time in the fresh air. Indeed if it had not been for the fact that he had previously led a different lifestyle in a totally different environment it is very unlikely that he would ever have developed this affliction. The shepherd loved his job and was only too well aware that it was largely this that was responsible for the fact that he had been able to keep his condition in check.

Many years ago my old friend Arthur Forster worked out a successful relaxation technique and with his kind permission I will conclude this chapter by sharing his advice with you.

The art of relaxation
Relaxation is an art, and like all skills it has to be learned. It is not easy, but everyone is capable of doing so and will obtain great benefit if they take the time and are determined. The few minutes each day that are required are a small price to pay for the great benefits that are obtained. Relaxed people are happier people, and thus are easier to live and work with. A relaxation period of

up to twenty minutes each day becomes a habit that is much looked forward to. Likewise, shorter periods taken when the opportunity arises — on the bus, or in the Underground, or even during the brief interval spent waiting for the traffic lights to change — take the sting out of the day. Relaxation simply means allowing the body to completely "flop" and to become "heavy" as you either lie on your couch or adapt to the situation in which you find yourself while relaxing. How is it achieved?

1. Choose the room in your house that is the quietest, and has a bed or couch on which you can stretch out completely and comfortably. This should be firm but not hard, and wide enough for you to lie on with both arms by your sides but not touching the body. You will need a small pillow and maybe a light covering. The light should be minimal and definitely not shining into your face. Pay a visit to the toilet beforehand, as an urgent call, or the need to go, can spoil your relaxation completely.

2. It is better if the body is not restricted by clothing that is even a little tight. An unclothed state is best but if this is not possible for any reason, then all tight clothing should be loosened as far as possible.

3. Lie on the bed or couch on your back. Leave a slight gap between your body and your arms, and open your legs slightly. This avoids skin sticking to skin and becoming uncomfortable. Air should be able to flow all round the body. The palms of the hands should be turned slightly uppermost, but without placing any strain on any muscle. This helps to prevent you clenching your fists. Make sure that your

body is straight — imagine a line passing through your nose, straight down the middle of your chest, and between your knees and ankles. Remember that you are going to stay still for some minutes, so be sure that you are comfortable.

The relaxation

Close your eyes, and begin to take long, deep breaths that reach to the depths of your lungs. Breathe out fully each time, while thinking of chasing the stale air from the deep areas of the lungs that many people never do get rid of. Count your breaths for a while.

Now turn your thoughts to your body and your desire to relax it completely.

1. Begin at your feet, and allow every muscle and tendon to simply let go. Wriggle your toes to begin with, then allow them to become still. Allow the whole foot to let go, and the muscles to relax. It will begin to feel heavy . . . remember that you have two feet, and let them both relax.

2. Now think of your calves and lower legs, allowing them to relax in the same manner. Continue up the legs to the thighs and hips, allowing them to begin feeling heavy, as if made of lead. They should feel as if they are about to fall through the couch. This is relaxation!

3. Continue the same procedure into the lower abdomen and the buttocks. This will bring you to the lower back. The whole spine should be allowed to sink onto the couch or bed until it is as straight as possible, and the big muscles of the back are released completely, as far up as the skull.

4. Take a moment to think of your arms, and make sure that they too are relaxed in every muscle right up to the shoulders.

5. Slightly open your mouth, and allow the facial muscles to relax fully. Do not forget the tongue. Let it "flop" in the mouth very loosely, and allow the eyelids to relax and avoid "fluttering". The muscles affecting the neck, jaws, and sides of the face should also be relaxed.

By now you should be feeling a great sense of well-being, almost one of levitation. Take a moment to check the state of your body — is every part comfortable? It should be, if you took the trouble to prepare yourself properly in the beginning. You will be completely and utterly relaxed. Getting to this stage should have taken about five minutes. It will take less time as you become practised in the art, until you can completely relax in only a few seconds.

Having made a physical check, you must empty the mind of all the worries and concerns of the day — the economics of the week, what you are having for your next meal, the remark that was made that upset you — all must be banished from the mind and thus from your relaxed body. To do this you must use your imagination and bring to mind a scene that you find pleasant, and to which only you are a witness. Then you should lie there and enjoy it. For example, think of a field of ripe corn, that stretches as far as you can see. You are drinking in the scene . . . the corn waving in the light summer breeze . . . the bright blue sky, with maybe a drifting cloud or two . . . the trees bordering the field . . . and the birds singing in them . . . the buttercups, poppies, daisies . . . and, if you are quiet enough, the rabbit that scampers around your feet. Take in this scene over and over again. Your body will respond, and much of the pain that you have been feeling will drift away — seemingly into your couch. Headaches, tired feet, backache, etc., will all ease.

Do not "time" your relaxation with a timer or a clock. Judge the time for yourself and accept that a minute can be a long time when you are waiting for it to pass. When you have been relaxing for ten, fifteen or twenty minutes, or what you are able to spare, gently begin to wake up your body — by wriggling the toes, the fingers, and easing the muscles back to activity. Having done this, rise from your bed or couch in the way you should get out of bed in the morning — or at any time. Turn onto your side, lift up your knees, lower your feet over the edge of the couch or bed, and gently lower them while pushing up at the same time on the underside of your arm, assisted by the upper arm, to an upright position. This method will avoid putting any strain on the spine.

Such a period of relaxation should be taken every day at least once. In a short time you will look forward to it, and you will make time for it. It becomes a part of life, like breakfast or your mid-morning tea. You will find that relaxation can be undertaken in all manner of situations as you become more adept at it. Minutes spent waiting for the dentist or osteopath can be spent in relaxation, with considerable benefit to the treatment to come. To become a relaxed person is to become a nicer person, and when you think of it, it is of excellent value because it costs nothing except a few minutes of your time.

5

Pneumonia

AT THE END of a very demanding and tiring lecture tour in South America I became slightly unwell. Fortunately, this is rather unusual for me because I am blessed with great health, good stamina and boundless energy. However, on this occasion I felt badly lacking in energy and altogether off-colour. I put it down to having had to travel by air to a different city every day for the changing venues of my lectures at the various universities where I had been scheduled to speak. I wasn't sorry to go home and arrived at the clinic to find a great many patients waiting. Although I only arrived back at three o'clock in the afternoon, I was back at work at four o'clock. Towards the end of the evening I became more and more unwell. I was coughing and generally I felt as if I had a bad dose of flu; nevertheless I had to put on a brave face.

The last patient that evening was not too easily fooled

as he was a practising physician himself. This gentleman was a well-known pathologist and after I had seen to him, he turned to me and asked me if I was feeling under the weather. I replied that he wasn't far off the mark. He then suggested that we turn the tables and when he climbed down from the treatment table he proposed that I climb up and he would check me over. He borrowed my stethoscope and, with a worried look on his face, he then told me that he suspected that I had pneumonia. I laughed at him and assumed that he must be exaggerating; nevertheless, I took his advice and retired immediately for the night. When I woke up I realised that he couldn't have been far wrong in his diagnosis as by this time I could not get out of bed. It was fortunate that no clinic had been scheduled for that day and by nine o'clock in the morning I decided to phone my best friend, who has been in medical practice for many years. This was quite a performance because he lives in the Netherlands whereas I reside in Scotland. However, after I had recited the symptoms to him, he asked me to cough over the telephone, to the great hilarity of my wife. He then confirmed the pathologist's diagnosis — pneumonia. This was my first personal encounter with the subject of this chapter.

It was obvious that immediate action had to be taken and I started taking large doses of Echinaforce, a natural antibiotic for which I have great regard and which I generally prescribe under similar circumstances. I took Echinaforce in combination with some other homoeopathic remedies, and I found that by lunchtime the following day my illness was on the turn. It wasn't a full recovery of course, as pneumonia is not shaken off so easily, but I realised that I was on the mend.

According to the book, pneumonia is an acute infection of the alveolar spaces of the lung. Of course there are many different manifestations of pneumonia and it also depends how we contract it. In my case it was probably the extremely heavy programme that had been scheduled for me, together with the daily travelling by plane, that caused my natural energies to become imbalanced. Anyway, to my friend it looked as if it was a viral pneumonia — with which I tended to agree — caused by a fairly common virus. With care and attention this virus can usually be overcome successfully.

If the pneumonia is caused by other kinds of infection, the effects on the lungs can be much more serious and certain respiratory infections can take over. In such cases careful medical attention and a sometimes lengthy period of convalescence are required. Antibiotics or other drugs are generally prescribed for this condition. However, I maintain that in these cases too it is still wise to use Echinaforce alongside other prescribed remedies, as this will help to relieve any congestion. I have treated many patients who have been prescribed penicillin or sulphonamides, and even then the benefits of Echinaforce could not be denied. Such patients should take complete bed rest and drink at least 10–12 pints of fluid daily. It is also important to make sure that the diet is kept very light and it should include some natural rice and plenty of blackcurrant juice. If the patient is in pain, I would also recommend the remedy Petaforce.

A more serious strain of pneumonia can be caused by a virus from the group A streptococci. In this case the symptoms can include tonsillitis, pharyngitis and flu-like conditions. Great care must be taken and most physicians will be fully aware of the seriousness of this illness and will give the patient his full support. Here again I would recommend Echinaforce, as well as Usneasan when the patient experiences excessive coughing. These two remedies can safely be taken alongside any allopathic drug prescribed by the physician.

47

There are several serious types of pneumonia and we should remember that if the illness is ignored and the patient does not take sufficient bed rest, the consequences could be most unpleasant. It must be said that cases of viral pneumonia seem to be more prevalent nowadays, especially in the big cities, and I can only think that the cause of this trend must lie in the environment. It is claimed, however, that there is no known cause of viral pneumonia, but in contrast to bacterial pneumonia its sudden onset and the symptoms of infection are mostly recognised in pulmonary symptoms. Coughs, breathlessness and headaches are often experienced and because of the accompanying throat irritation it is important to choose the appropriate remedies.

Old-fashioned remedies often prove to be of great help when suffering from pneumonia. For example, gargling with 0.5 per cent hydrogen peroxide. The patient should be careful not to swallow this solution, but just gargle with it. Chamomile tea can be used, as a drink or for gargling, and this will also help to ease the throat irritation. Then there is a most unusual remedy called Molkosan, which is available from Bioforce. In Switzerland this liquid is popularly used as a salad dressing, but as this remedy consists of milk whey, it contains strong antiseptic properties and serves us well as a gargle. I would heartily recommend Molkosan for all kinds of pneumonia, as well as for other throat or cough problems. For over thirty years now Molkosan has been a good friend to me whenever throat infections have had to be overcome. It is true that whey possesses antibiotic properties, but it is less well known that it is also useful for promoting the circulation to the liver, reducing the cholesterol level and detoxifying of the bowels. Whey obtained from sheep's milk can sometimes be even better and I have prescribed this for some extremely persistent cases of pneumonia.

If the pneumonia patient's condition is highly toxic, it will be important to detoxify the body as quickly and thoroughly as possible. It is often thought that the cause of pneumonia is a germ or a virus, but it is more often the result of a tired, imbalanced condition, as was the case with me. For this reason we must pay attention to our immune system and ensure that we take sufficient care of it. In the orthodox treatment of pneumonia, when sometimes excessive quantities of antibiotics are used to eliminate the superficial germ or virus, the underlying cause is not removed and it is easy to become complacent because of a rapid improvement. The patient may be adversely affected by a short- or long-term course of antibiotics and other problems may result. Molkosan, or the use of natural yoghurt or acidophilus, is important when antibiotics are encouraged to destroy the bacteria, including many of the defensive bacteria in the bowels. With a recurrent problem of lung disease and the suppression of the relevant symptoms, the possibility of developing more serious problems, even to the extent of lung cancer, cannot be disregarded.

It is very important when one is prone to pneumonia to take good care of the dietary regime and in this respect I must reiterate that fasting can never cause any harm, as long as plenty of fluids are taken. Always try to avoid milk and dairy products wherever possible. This advice may appear to contradict my recommendation that the patient use Molkosan, but for this purpose Molkosan is not classified alongside other dairy products. Fruit juices are extremely beneficial, although I would suggest a limit to the amount of orange juice. I would rather see the patient drink more pineapple, blackcurrant or rosehip juices and some herbal teas. Some simple water treatments may also be helpful; details of suitable ones to try can be found in my book *Water — Healer or Poison?* Water, assuming that it is of an acceptable quality, is an ideal agent in the cleansing process to help the body rid itself of toxicity.

It is worth remembering that herbalism holds many remedies and cures. For example, you may freely use watercress (*Nasturtium officinale*) — which contains chlorophyll and is also rich in calcium, vitamin C and mustard oils. These ingredients combine to make watercress a tremendous antibiotic, and one that has a very beneficial influence on the flora in the bowels. I would also wholeheartedly recommend East Indian cress (*Tropaeolum majus*); although this plant used to be regarded primarily as an ornamental variety, it is rich in benzyl mustard oils. It has great disinfectant properties, especially on the mucous membranes and on the throat, and the fact that the remedial effects can be obtained by chewing the leaves makes it more attractive as a herbal remedy. Especially for emphysema, bronchitis and pneumonia the above-mentioned remedies will usually prove effective and they can all be used in combination with *Imperatoria*. Never forget that nature is on our side and readily supplies us with simple remedies that can help us to overcome some very serious conditions.

6

Asthmatic Conditions

YEARS BEFORE I was ever called upon to treat the many, many patients with asthmatic conditions I have examined during my medical career, I had already come into contact with asthma whilst at primary school. This goes way back to the Second World War when it became clear that a young and close relative was suffering from a chronic bronchial asthmatic condition. She was a regular visitor to our home and whenever she suffered an attack I would try and comfort her. As young as I was, I will never forget my feeling of helplessness when I saw this young girl suffering. Many a time the doctor would have to be called out when she suffered a severe attack. I would pray very hard as there was little else I could do. I was very fond of her, and I suffered with her during these sudden attacks.

It was not only the severity, but the suddenness of these attacks that was so frightening. For no apparent reason the wheezing would start and it seemed that there was little we could do to stop this developing into a full-blown attack. It never seemed to matter what action she did or didn't take — the attack would just run its course. Relief eventually came for the poor girl when her parents were able to send her to Switzerland with the help of some money that was collected. She went to Davos and in the clear mountain air she appeared to fare much better. However, on returning to the damp atmosphere of her home town, she became as bad as ever again. Eventually, it was decided to perform an operation and this has had to be repeated several times in order to save her life. Thank goodness, science has progressed considerably since then, but I often regret that at the time I was too young to be of any real help to her, because I now know that nature could have helped in many ways to relieve the condition she suffered from so severely.

There are several kinds of asthma, but a bronchial asthma can be very nasty indeed. It is a condition that manifests itself by recurrent paroxysms of dyspnoea of the wheezing type caused by narrowing of the smaller bronchi and bronchioles. This condition is often hereditary, although in our family no real indication of this could be found. Looking back at her condition and knowing what I know now, I feel that this young girl must have had an allergic constitution. Because of the circumstances we were living under, especially during the war years, it would not have been easy to overcome this, even if we had known about it at the time. However, I can assure you that her condition was eventually brought under control. She subsequently married and her children do not appear to have inherited any asthmatic tendencies.

The asthmatic condition, which is one of three major lung diseases, is often extremely confusing for those who are afflicted by it, because the causes can be so diverse. An attack may come on either at night or in the early morning, and shortage of breath is experienced, making the sufferer gasp for air, trying to gulp and force this air into the chest. Such an attack can last for several hours, and can return at sporadic or frequent intervals. Thus the asthmatic patient can hardly fail to become more and more uptight and nervous. We categorise this state as nervous asthma.

This condition was clearly apparent in another young girl, who became more tense and uptight about her condition during her teenage years. She wondered and worried whether she would ever be able to find herself a boyfriend who would be prepared to put up with her condition. Fortunately, she is now happily married and has learned through experience to keep her tense nature in check with some of the relaxation exercises I have taught her. She no longer panics and her asthmatic problem has been stabilised since I discovered an underlying allergic condition. In fact, this young mother has very few health problems indeed.

Nevertheless, when we look for the reason why these little tubes constrict the breathing in this way, we must conclude that no satisfactory answer has yet been found. At least one in every hundred persons used to suffer from asthmatic tendencies and this proportion is increasing steadily. I participate on a regular basis in a radio programme with the well-known broadcaster Gloria Hunniford, who is patron of the London Chest Hospital, and I have been astounded to find out how many people phone in with questions about asthma during these broadcasts. Unfortunately, the general input is that many of them had never previously experienced such problems, yet now they have been diagnosed as having asthmatic complaints. It appears that in Britain at the moment, in localised areas, asthmatic conditions have become almost epidemic. With this feedback we must come to the conclusion that the occurrence of asthma is definitely on the increase. To my mind there can be no doubt that factors such as atmospheric conditions, air pollution, acid rain and, above all, a less effective immune system, are taking their toll. Although asthma is generally considered to be an illness that strikes the younger generation and often clears during or after puberty, I am worried about the apparent increase in asthma affecting adults, which leads me to wonder even more what the cause might be.

We can take our pick of possible causes that could be at the root of the problem. The development of asthma can be influenced by the environment, the weather, or any kind of allergy — for example to one or more food items, pets, washing powder or perfume. I am often baffled to see that such problems can sometimes disappear as suddenly as they arose, while in other cases they continue with the same severity, despite the individual having taken certain measures. The circumstances that can trigger off an asthma attack could be as seemingly insignificant as being in the same room as a small canary in a cage. Given these factors, it is my belief that the ability to pinpoint certain allergies can play a significant part in detecting the possible causes of an asthma attack. In the next chapter I will discuss the subject of allergies in greater detail.

It is often more difficult to identify the psychological factors relating to asthma, though these can have a considerable bearing on the condition. I have indeed known patients whose asthmatic attacks became a thing of the past when their circumstances changed, or a specific incident occurred which proved that the condition had a nervous origin.

An example of this can be found in the remarkable story I read in a book by Martin Koje. He wrote about an asthmatic patient who arrived at his hotel late in the evening. Immediately upon his arrival he went to bed and fell sound asleep. In the dark of the night he suddenly awoke realising that he had forgotten to open the window. He immediately felt an asthma attack coming on and in his panic he stormed over to the window, which he was unable to open, and bashed away at it until he broke the glass. He breathed in the fresh air, returned to bed, and continued to sleep soundly until the next morning — when his cure came. He then realised that he had not broken the window, but instead had demolished a mirror which had shown him a reflection of the moon and which in his panic he had imagined to be the window. This anecdote shows that the mind is stronger than the body. In no way would I dare to suggest that asthma is always a psychological problem, but over the years I have seen, especially with patients whose asthma flares up during times of tension, that if the patient is encouraged to think more positively, the treatment will prove to be so much more successful.

The great secret of improvement lies in the fact that the patient trusts the practitioner's judgement, but equally important is the fact that the patient sincerely wishes to be cured. This may appear a controversial statement, but on reflection its truth will become clear. Many a patient who has lived with an asthmatic condition for some time will have decided that he or she will just have to learn to live with it. However, it is very important that they firmly believe that this condition can be overcome and they should dedicate themselves to that end. I can promise you that I have seen determination pay off. Never give up hope, because much can be done to overcome asthma.

Asthmatic patients who tend to panic and become nervous would do well to understand that the key to recovery is often hidden within that person. Try and learn how to relax; to this end some of the relaxation exercises outlined elsewhere in this book will come in useful. When you are troubled by worries, particularly emotional worries, look for someone to confide in who might be able to help you solve them. I have often seen misunderstandings in a marriage trigger off an attack in an asthma patient. In one case I treated a male patient who suffered from very severe attacks of asthma. Eventually, the cause of his condition was traced back to the dictatorial manner of his wife. After his wife died, the poor man's health seemed to improve by leaps and bounds. It was not because he had not been fond of his wife, but the oppressive attitude with which his wife had run the home had taken its toll. I learned that at all times he had to take off his shoes when entering the house, and after having worked in the garden she would carefully check that he had not brought any dirt into the house on his clothing. Her overly house-proud attitude had made him so tense that his asthmatic condition had steadily worsened. After the death of his wife he became a different person, which was a sad reflection on their marital relationship.

Similarly I have often seen the reverse of this with female patients, whose husbands may be alcoholics, workaholics, or sports fanatics who take little or no interest in them or their family. The wife feels herself and rest of the family to be ignored and taken for granted, and the tension that results may well bring on an attack. One such case comes to mind concerning a woman who was treated like a piece of the furniture by her overbearing husband. Her asthmatic problems had shown no signs of improvement and yet in my mind I was convinced that my diagnosis had been correct and that it was her husband that was the obstacle to any improvement. After I had done everything possible for her, I asked to speak to her husband. I gave him the facts and asked him to take her out for a meal sometimes and spend some time with her and show her some consideration. I told him that I felt sure that both he and his wife would be repaid in ways they hadn't dreamed of. In front of me is a letter I received from that particular lady some time later:

"Thank you so much for what you have done for us. My husband and I are now the proud parents of a baby boy. The birth went very well, my asthma is under control and even during labour I never had an asthma attack. Life is very sweet and totally different to what I experienced before I attended your clinic."

How marvellous it is to lose a patient in this way. It proves how important it is, especially if the patient is of a nervous disposition, that he or she receives all possible help and support. Therefore, be determined to clear away all obstacles and replace them with positive suggestions, followed by the appropriate remedies. Practise some breathing and relaxation exercises, try and loosen all the muscles and ligaments, while telling yourself to be completely at peace. Especially during an attack, open and close the eyes ten times, try and breathe slowly — in and out, in and out — while telling yourself to keep calm and that nothing can disturb you. Feeling totally relaxed with the aid of some of the breathing and tension-relieving methods mentioned in this book will help to stave off some of these dreaded attacks.

The Hara breathing method is also recommended for asthmatic patients. Always remember that it is possible for the patient to exert a great deal of control with relatively simple methods.

Now let's look at asthma as a condition. Sometimes we hear from patients that it all started with a throat or chest infection that appeared to settle in and has since become chronic. It may have been a sinus infection or a tonsil or adenoid problem and out of the blue they experience a severe asthma attack. We can then only conclude that the mucosa of the bronchi have thickened and that congestion has resulted, causing wheezing. Unless more serious problems also exist, everything possible should be done to relieve the congestion. Many people seem to disbelieve, mistakenly, that asthma can be found written on death certificates as the actual cause of death. Many non-sufferers regard it as a mere inconvenience and know little more about it than it concerns breathing difficulties. The *Hertfordshire Mercury* of 7 December carried the following interesting article:

Dramatic increase in asthma "road" deaths
Choked roads may be claiming the lives of a whole new group of "victims" — asthma sufferers.

There has been a staggering 54 per cent rise in deaths from the condition.

East Herts health authority's director of public health Irene Clarke believes the big increase could be related to fumes emitted from the huge rise in traffic on the area's roads — which in turn shows a 40 per cent increase over the past ten years.

The figures contained in the authority's annual health report disclose that there were ten deaths last year and thirteen the year before.

The area's hospitals are finding that they are dealing with far more cases of asthma in their chest clinics than ever before.

The report reveals that the rises in cases are particularly high in the Broxbourne and Welwyn/Hatfield areas. "These districts are closely associated with the M25 and A1(M) respectively," says Dr Clarke. She emphasises: "These disturbing figures suggest that it is time that the issue of public transport was re-examined not only because of the political instability in the Middle East, but also because of the mental stress created in the outer London area by excessive traffic density."

Dr Clarke told the *Mercury* that at present there were only "weak" statistical reasons for suggesting a link between the illness and traffic increase — but it was thought it could well be a "contributory factor".

Congestion is so often the topic of letters I receive from people, and as asthma can definitely be fatal, it most certainly justifies attention. Congestion could even result from a relatively minor catarrhal condition of the nose. I don't want to unduly alarm my readers, but if minor problems are noticed, these must be interpreted as the body telling us that something must be done. At this stage some simple action may ward off further complications.

Take, for example, the mother who breastfeeds her baby in the knowledge that mother's milk contains all the essential digestive enzymes. When weaning the baby and introducing it to cow's milk, it is not uncommon to encounter problems such as infantile eczema or asthmatic complications. We then wonder what is happening. I personally feel that the problems are caused by the fact that cow's milk contains nine times more protein than breast milk, and the digestive system of the little one cannot cope with this enormous change. Allergy problems may well result, so please spare a thought for the poor baby who is being bombarded with the extra protein, which burns much more slowly than, for instance, carbohydrates. It is not surprising that problems can then arise. The extra mucus formed from dairy products is another result. So often these little signs are not correctly interpreted, yet these symptoms are like alarm bells set into action by the body, indicating that it cannot cope.

A number of remedies can help get rid of the congestion, apart from a change in dietary management, and I often prescribe Uneasan sometimes backed up by Echinaforce to act as an antibiotic. It is not enough to suppress asthmatic conditions with drugs, whilst ignoring the underlying cause. The cause must be investigated and located in order to determine the correct treatment. Once this has been done the rest will usually fall into place. Under these circumstances we may choose to undergo tests to determine any unusual sensitivities or allergies in order to discover the way to recovery.

In the case of allergic asthmatic problems it will be helpful to use the old-fashioned remedy kelp, and to this end I would recommend Kelpasan tablets. Kelpasan is made from pure sea algae from the Pacific Ocean and contains all the recommended trace elements. Four tablets taken first thing in the morning with a glass of hot water will often clear some of the allergic reactions. If these reactions are very severe, you can also take some *Harpagophytum*, which acts as a helpful agent to counter many general allergies.

Such remedies may also be used in the treatment of infected asthma, but I would rather recommend Pollinosan, which is another excellent remedy from the Bioforce range. I will say more about this remedy in a later chapter on hay fever. Although it is essentially designed to treat that allergy, it is also beneficial in cases of infected asthma.

In cases of cardiac asthma extra care must be taken and fortunately, and rightly so, most cardiac asthmatic patients are under the constant care of their general practitioner. Here again, as with all asthmatic conditions, it is important to take care of the immune system and therefore to pay attention to nutrition. I will conclude this chapter with a recommended diet, which has been specially designed for asthmatic conditions (see pages 70–71).

As I have said before, there are many causes of asthmatic conditions and it is not only the cat, the dog or the canary that can trigger off a sudden attack, they may be caused by some very serious infections, such as the *Streptococcus pneumoniae* or the *Streptococcus pyoginis*, or even the *Haemophilus influenzae*. Hereditary conditions can play a part and although studies have indicated that for about 40 per cent of asthmatic patients the cause may be related to allergic infections, I believe that the time has come for this data to be revised in the light of atmospheric influences, which appear to be a significant cause of asthmatic conditions. Nowadays it seems that almost all age groups are much more likely to be affected by asthma than in the past. This fact presents us with a totally different situation to that which we have been used to, and it causes great worry for an asthmatic patient who appears so helpless during an attack.

Sometimes I decide to give a patient acupuncture treatment, which gives great relief during an asthma attack. At the same time I will take an ice-cold cloth or an ice cube and place this on the ninth dorsal vertebra, a measure that usually provides immediate relief. Physiotherapy is also of great help to an asthma patient.

The body needs plenty of oxygen and in order to provide a constant supply the alveoli are supposed to effect an interchange between oxygen and carbon dioxide. The total size of the lungs is estimated to be about 90 m^2 — forty times as much as the total skin surface. A total of 4.5 litres, or nine pints, of blood circulate constantly through the lungs. The lungs are normally very elastic and they are enclosed within a thin "bag" with a double wall. The outside wall of the chest tissue is called the pleura paritalis, and where the air tubes and lungs meet each other, i.e. the inner wall of this bag, the pleura viceralis encloses both the lungs. The air pressure within the lungs relates to the external atmospheric pressure. Because the lungs have a tendency to close there exists a power that dictates the pressure to the lung tissue, making sure that the pressure to both tissues decreases. This pressure ensures that the lungs do not collapse. Every time we breathe in, new air will be supplied. This is an active process where the breathing muscles pull the ribs to expand the chest area. Some of the ribs are movable, but other ribs, especially the second to seventh rib, go up and down with our breathing, which is another reason why breathing exercises are very important.

The spine also plays a great part in this process, hence the reason why qualified osteopathic treatment is so conducive to creating room to breathe more easily. This explains why so many asthma patients benefit greatly from osteopathic treatment. The super-efficient co-operation between heart and lungs will ensure that there is an efficient supply of oxygen. It is interesting to see that during each inhalation and exhalation cycle only 15 per cent of the total lung volume is interchanged. Physiologists therefore often use a spirometer to register the amount of air exhaled. They have determined that a man weighing approximately 70 kg uses 300 cm^3 oxygen per minute and that as a result of the metabolic processes 220 cm^3 of carbon dioxide is produced. About half of all the air inhaled reaches the alveoli and it is there that the air is in close contact with the blood and the breathing centre receives constant and up-to-date information on the tension in the lung tissue and the breathing muscles. This is a very important source of information and in order for the system to work efficiently, breathing exercises, physiotherapy and often acupuncture can be extremely helpful. With this knowledge we will understand why smokers experience so much more difficulty, as the system is labouring and working overtime to overcome the adverse effects of nicotine. It also explains why, in order to let this system work freely and happily, the patient has to try and avoid colds and other respiratory infections. Thus, by trying to ensure the most positive circumstances possible, a general improvement of the breathing function can be achieved.

The drugs that are used in the treatment of asthma are often of the antispasmodic variety and it would be sensible to investigate the alternatives that homoeopathic treatment has to offer. Homoeopathic principles are based on the formula of "like cures like", which was first put forward or, more correctly, rediscovered by Dr Samuel Hahnemann. This system has been developed into a complete medical treatment method over the years. Hahnemann was unhappy with the action of allopathic drugs. He tried the drug *Cinchona* on himself and was amazed to discover that it produced in him the very same symptoms of the disease it was supposed to cure. He repeated the experiments by using different drugs on other volunteers and his findings led to the confirmation of the great healing principle once pronounced by Paracelsus: *"simula similibus curentur"*. Remedies that were diluted one part in one hundred, more than thirty times, became commonplace in homoeopathic prescriptions, but this led to ridicule from allopathic doctors and "conventional" scientists. They claimed that the potency of the original substance could not possibly be significant in such a diluted solution. However, advocates of homoeopathy were not so ignorant as to be unaware of this possibility, but they maintained that a healing force was unlocked when a substance was succussed and diluted, giving homoeopathic remedies the capability of activating the healing process that is inherent in most of us. We frequently see evidence of this with asthma patients if they use *Arsen. alb.* D6–D30, *Nux vomica* D6–D20, *Zincum valerianicum* D3 or a high potency of *Belladonna*.

Cardiac asthma patients have a cardiac weakness and it is sometimes helpful to use the remedy Convascillan or some other *Convallaria* combination based on that lovely flower, the lily of the valley. Sometimes symptoms indicate the use of tissue salts like *Kali. phos.*, *Magnesium phos.*, *Nat. mur.*, *Calcium phos.*, or *Nat. sulph.* Herbal treatment should also be considered. I favour several combinations for the treatment of such conditions, but as I have already said, I would probably prescribe Echinaforce.

In congested conditions it is wise to use Bronchosan, which is a wonderful remedy for bronchial asthma and bronchitis. This, together with the Drosinula syrup, is usually of great help. I often prescribe Santasapina, a cough syrup which fortifies and strengthens the respiratory tract, especially during a period of increased danger of contagion and during cold weather. Coughs, hoarseness and inflammation of the mucous membranes are greatly relieved by taking Santasapina. It strengthens the body's defences by natural means and its honey content promotes the loosening of the tough mucus when coughing.

Asthma drops can only be prescribed by a physician and for certain conditions these can be extremely effective. They consist of a fresh herb preparation designed for the treatment of bronchial asthma and they work as an antispasmodic.

Chamomile is also a much-used herb and is suitable for many purposes. For chest conditions I would suggest that it be used as an infusion. Add one heaped teaspoon to half a pint of water and leave it to steep for a short while. Good results are obtained from an inhalation of chamomile, especially when it is used together with Poho oil. The same can be said about coltsfoot — *Tussilago farfara* — which is another remedy that is frequently recommended for asthma, pneumonia and bronchitis. To make a coltsfoot infusion add one heaped teaspoon of the flowers to half a pint of boiling water and leave it to infuse for ten minutes. The fresh juice can also be extracted from the flowers and this can be used as a tincture, to be diluted as desired. *Plantago lanceolata* is of great help when the lungs are painful, and this remedy may be used alongside any other kind of treatment. A variety of aromatic herbs such as thyme, marjoram, pine, lavender, eucalyptus or rosemary are not only pleasant to use, but also highly beneficial. In addition, asthmatic patients should never forget to use calcium to help maintain the tone and elasticity of the muscles.

I am often quizzed about my reasons for prescribing oil of evening primrose. This product is a panacea for many health complaints, among them bronchitis and asthma. The essential fatty acids contained in oil of evening primrose are very important as a nutrient and these cannot be produced inside the body, but are digested through the intake of food. As many people lack a sufficient supply of essential fatty acids, I often prescribe oil of evening primrose as a food supplement. Essential fatty acids are an integral component of the chemical messengers known as prostaglandins, which are hormone-like substances that control different metabolic pathways.

One of the most important of such messengers is the prostaglandin PGE1, as this controls many of the body functions. Essential fatty acids are all unsaturated but before they can be metabolised to form prostaglandins we have to be encouraged to eat more unsaturated fatty acids, such as gammalinoleic acid or GLA, a precursor of PGE1. This process may sometimes be inefficient, so a dietary source of GLA may prove useful. Breast milk is one of the best known sources of correctly balanced EFA and GLA, and experts have for a long time tried, to no effect, to find a more convenient source. The evening primrose plant is now universally acknowledged as one of the richest natural sources of GLA from which the body produces many of the vital prostaglandins, and its oil is now recognised as one of the standard GLA and EFA food supplements. Nature's Best's evening primrose is encapsulated with gelatin, glycerin and purified water and for the conditions I am concerned with in this book I can wholeheartedly recommend this supplement.

The same goes for royal jelly. I sometimes think back to 1960 when Dr Vogel and I were working together in the first naturopathic clinic in the Netherlands. Even at that time Dr Vogel had already decided to utilise a royal jelly preparation and had been prescribing this with great results to his patients. There is no doubt that royal jelly possesses biological qualities of the highest quality, for it enables the queen bee to lay as many as 2,000 eggs daily — and this with a single fertilisation. This is an amazing example of natural fertility and this biological achievement cannot be found in any other living creature. Dr Vogel acclaimed the benefits of royal jelly at the Second International Biogenetic Congress under the chairmanship of Dr Daleazzi, who read most of the paper dealing with the research findings on royal jelly. In this paper it was pointed out how royal jelly rejuvenates through the endocrine glands and how successful this combination was for asthma and bronchitis patients. Royal jelly must be considered as one of the very best prophylactic measures that exist.

While taking all this advice to heart, let us make sure that the patient obtains plenty of fresh air. He or she must try to relax, take plenty of rest, keep warmly dressed and, finally, ensure that good care is taken to follow a balanced diet. I am sometimes met with ridicule or a sceptical attitude when I insist on the importance of better dietary management. Let me assure you of the benefits of a correct diet in relation to the conditions we are concerned with. Of course, it must be true that the food we eat affects our body in many ways and therefore that the assimilation of nutrients and the elimination needed to purify the body is totally dependent on our food intake. Nutrition is always important, not only because of the effects of deficiencies in vitamins, minerals or trace elements, but also in view of the allergic reactions that can be caused by poor dietary habits or an excess of food. I have already mentioned some of the foods to avoid and in the next chapter, which discusses allergies, I will provide more detailed guidelines. If a balanced diet is followed and the condition still does not improve, then a stricter diet may be necessary. In this case the diet should consist mainly of fresh fruit and fresh juices, including salads, honey, nuts, herbal teas and only a limited amount of meat. No dairy products whatsoever should be taken, except yoghurt, which has the correct acid content, or milk whey obtained from either cow's or sheep's milk.

We see all too often what a crucial role the diet plays when an asthma patient experiences considerable improvement when dairy products have been eliminated from the diet, or another source of allergy has been pinpointed and acted upon. It also makes sense to take a supplement when it appears that vitamins, minerals, trace elements or other nutritional substances are lacking in the diet. Below is a translation of an article published on 13 June 1989 in a Dutch newspaper, the *Nieuwe Rotterdamse Courant:*

Do neuropeptides play a role in the origin of asthma?

It appears that two in every hundred people suffer from bronchial asthma, but it is undisputed that recently a great many more people have been bothered by hay fever. Yet the origins of these related conditions have not been fully discovered. The respiratory canals of bronchial asthma patients react with excessive speed to irritations which would not affect "normal" people. Serious anxiety is the result. Various substances in the inhaled air can act as irritants (allergens), of which pollen, plant spores, housemite, pets' hairs, etc. are well known and recognised as such. However, in research often no specific factors are discovered. Sometimes the cause is job-related, such as an asthmatic condition common to bakers. Whatever the cause, a respiratory sensitivity is present in the bronchi, i.e. the branches of the trachea or the windpipe. Similarly in hay fever such a sudden allergic reaction is not uncommon. For hay fever, please read allergic rhinitis (i.e. allergic nasal infection), as no hay is involved, nor fever. It is in fact pollen which causes the watery and swollen eyes and the weeping nose.

At the root of all these symptoms are defensive cells in the mucous membranes, which in the case of oversensitivity and contact with allergens react by discharging locally active substances, i.e. mediators, of which histamine is the most common. This substance causes contractions of the small, smooth muscles around the bronchi, resulting in extreme anxiety or shortage of breath. Histamine also stimulates an increased discharge through the mucous glands and a discharge of fluids from the defensive cells through the small capillaries, causing further narrowing of the respiratory tracts. These symptoms are present in anybody to whom histamine is supplied with the use of an aerosol, but in bronchial asthma patients the reaction is very much stronger and speedier, due to bronchial over-sensitivity.

Some Australian researchers now claim to have come up with an explanation for this excessive sensitivity. With immunocytochemical techniques they have been able to select certain interactive substances in the nerve fibres of the lung tissue. The nerve fibres influence the muscle tension, glandular secretion and veins. As well as stimulating fibres there are also fibres which act with a restraining influence. Neuropeptide VIP (vasoactive intestinal polypeptide) acts as an interactive substance between restraining fibres and bronchial muscles. In the Australian research it has been deduced that VIP is present in the nerve fibres of smooth muscle tissue, veins and the mucous membranes of "normal" cases. This, however, is not present in the lung tissue of asthmatic patients.

It has been known for a few years now that VIP is able to alleviate the severity of bronchial sensitivity. It has also been proved that VIP is capable of widening the bronchi. Therefore the research team concludes that bronchial asthma is caused by the non-presence of VIP, as the histamine effect is not curbed.

This conclusion, however, still does not supply us with a solution to the problem. The non-presence of VIP could be caused by an inherent or acquired synthesis disturbance, but it could also be lost as a result of the illness process.

Considering the above I am a fervent believer that a well-balanced diet can be conducive to overcoming asthmatic conditions and the following diet has been carefully worked out and is recommended for most asthma, hay fever, rhinitis and sinusitis cases.

Recommended diet for asthma, hay fever, rhinitis and sinusitis patients

Breakfast:

Grapefruit or unsweetened grapefruit juice.

Compote of apple, prunes and blackberries.

Porridge served with molasses or honey and soya milk or prune juice.

Cereal, such as muesli or oats mixed with equal parts of soya milk and watery apple juice, sweetened with molasses and water or prune juice.

Rye crispbread.

Wholemeal toast — no more than three times a week.

Lunch:

Salad, including most fresh vegetables and fruit except oranges.

Alfalfa seed sprouts, onions, garlic and grated carrots.

Vegetable soup, using Plantaforce as stock.

Rye crispbread or wholemeal bread.

Jacket potato, brown rice or barley, millet and potato, buckwheat.

Dinner:

Lamb — no more than twice a week.

Poultry, beef or rabbit — no more than once a week.

Any fresh sea fish — no more than twice a week.

Pulses, such as soya beans or tofu, aduki, kidney or haricot beans, lentils or chickpeas — to be included in at least two meals a week.

Fresh cooked vegetables, sea vegetables and bean sprouts.

A salad every day.

Potato or wholegrains, e.g. brown rice, barley, millet and/or potato, buckwheat, served with soya sauce or apple sauce.

Fruit.

Beverages:

China, Earl Grey, peppermint or rosehip tea without milk or sugar.

Bottled water.

Fruit juices, especially blackcurrant or pineapple juice.

Dressings, oils and condiments:

Dress salads with lemon juice or olive oil and lemon juice or cider vinegar. Flavour the dressings with garlic and herbs. No mayonnaise. The best oils to use are sunflower, soya or olive. Use plenty of herbs, especially sage, thyme, parsley and rosemary. Use Herbamare or Trocomare salt.

Foods to avoid:

Completely avoid all cow's milk dairy products, i.e. cheese, milk, skimmed milk, butter, etc. Avoid any kind of pork, whether it be bacon, ham or sausages. Avoid oranges, eggs, red wine, excessive tea, coffee and fatty foods. Reduce the intake of bread and wheat products, sugar and processed foods. Avoid common salt.

In the next chapter we look at allergies, but more information on this subject can be found in my book *Viruses, Allergies and the Immune System*.

7

Allergies

ALTHOUGH I HAVE written widely on the subject of allergies in my book *Viruses, Allergies and the Immune System*, I would like to delve a little deeper into some of the possible connections between allergies and the conditions described elsewhere in this book.

In today's society much publicity is given to the subject of allergies and numerous therapists have found this a lucrative field; many people have gone from one to the other for advice, spending a great deal of money, while eventually being no better off in terms of their health. Therefore I would like to explain some of the naturopathic views on this subject. A naturopath is trained to look for the underlying cause of any illness and will not over-emphasise the importance of the allergy as such. Over the years I have seen many allergic reactions disappear when I had treated the immune system on a naturopathic basis. This has encouraged me to approach the allergy problem in the established naturopathic way, i.e. advising the patients to improve their dietary management and obtain plenty of sunlight, fresh air and rest. In some cases these measures alone may prove effective, but unfortunately not in every case.

Today the naturopath has to look for ways to help the immune system without the risk of side-effects in order to overcome allergies. With allergic reactions we look for causes that create such an unpleasant response and in this respect we have learned much from research into hay fever. In this category we will specifically look at house mite, certain kinds of fruit, shellfish and dairy products. There are quite a number of things that could trigger off an allergic reaction. It could easily be animals, sugar, wheat, cheese or chocolate that is the cause of such a reaction, and those reactions are often due to hypersensitivity.

An allergic reaction need not always be a violent response, but even if relatively mild, these reactions may be the cause of urticaria (nettle rash), oedema, breathing problems, asthmatic conditions, incontinence or a variety of other physical manifestations. If severe allergic reactions are experienced we sometimes see symptoms of fever or in some cases a tendency to faint.

It is the task of our immune system to protect us and we often see that if our immunity is impaired in any way or for whichever reason, certain allergic reactions may appear. There are, of course, a number of ways to find out more about our allergic tendencies. There is the well-known skin prick test, as well as blood tests, hair tests, elimination therapy, and quite a few more ways in which allergies can be pinpointed. From experience, I doubt if any of these tests are always accurate, or at any rate sufficiently so to give us a true picture. But let me say that I consider it unwise to run from one allergy clinic to another. This is more likely to cause confusion, if for no other reason than that the immune system, for all its wonderful actions, is not always easy to follow. The immune system changes very frequently and even immunologists find it difficult to ascertain exactly how it works.

I remember a mother who, before she came to my clinic for advice, had taken .her daughter to three different allergy clinics and each time she had been given a different diagnosis and was advised accordingly. After each consultation she eliminated the relevant nutritional substances, until I was obliged to diagnose that the girl was suffering from scurvy due to malnutrition. Who would have believed it could be possible in this day and age? This example goes to show that allergy testing must be handled very carefully and I am sure that in many cases the allergy could have been detected with some simple dietary experiments.

In the *Dictionary of Nutrition and Food Technology*, compiled by Professor A. Bender, we can read that "an allergy is an altered or abnormal tissue reaction which may be caused by contact between a foreign protein, the allergen and sensitive body tissues". This is a statement of pure common sense and it is armed with common sense that we have to tackle the allergic reaction that triggers off bronchial and asthmatic conditions. Professor Bender also believes that food allergies are most common in infants and that the usual causes are eggs, milk and wheat. Reactions may include urticaria, hay fever, asthma and dyspepsia.

One of the most frequent questions put to me in radio programmes and lectures is: "Can air pollution be the cause of allergies and can this result in an asthmatic or related condition?" It is true that we all breathe in the same air. The great difference lies in where exactly we are living — and I am certain that the Chernobyl incident is bound to have its effects in Great Britain, as it will in the heart of Africa. The atmospheric conditions where we live, whether they be dry or damp, are also significant. If we suffer from a catarrhal condition and the oxygen supply is poor, then we may become allergic to certain conditions. The possibility of a less effective immune system, owing to a deterioration in the quality of the three forms of energy essential to the survival of mankind, namely water, food and air, needs to be considered and the better we protect ourselves, e.g. by taking supplementary vitamins, minerals and trace elements, the less oxygen our body actually needs. One of the reasons that the old naturopathic treatment used to be so successful was because our ancestors not only enjoyed cleaner air and a more natural diet, but it is also safe to assume that their food was of a higher nutritional value, because of the richer supplies of vitamins, minerals and trace elements present in the soil. Fertilisation was done by natural means in those days. Oxygen is important and will contribute to minimising allergies because it has the ability to fight any disease. Unfortunately, in our present environment even the quality of the oxygen supply is diminishing, as the plankton in the world's seas — our greatest source of oxygen and so essential for the health of mankind — is slowly rotting away. This is a result of all the rubbish we are dumping into the seas.

Is all this, then, the reason that degenerative diseases are becoming so much more prevalent? Is it true that, for instance, cancer is not a disease but a lengthy degenerative process? No matter what, we must protect ourselves against the bacterial and viral invaders and in this oxygen is one of our great allies. Let us also remember that our lungs in themselves are a great eliminator. They instinctively recognise and dispose of carbon dioxide, the waste product from breathing, also the carbonic acid which is stored in the tissues, affecting the metabolic system. With this in mind it may be worth pointing out that nettles are known for their effectiveness in clearing waste material from the body and just in case you didn't know, nettle soup makes a really healthy and tasty dish.

Another increasing source of allergies nowadays is that common nutritional substance known as wheat. A wheat allergy can display itself in unpleasant skin complaints, wheezing and other such breathing problems. Why is it that a product as common as wheat can cause such dire problems? I think the answer must lie in the artificial processing of the wheat grain. Throughout the world, wherever wheat is grown organically, allergic reactions to this cereal are unknown. Unfortunately in our affluent society such reactions are a growing problem and it only takes a simple test to prove that wheat is the cause of many allergies.

There is a tendency to attack such allergies aggressively, but this is unwise as this may cause unexpected side-effects. Allergies should be tackled with common sense and this brings me back to the fact that naturopathy offers us a very acceptable and totally safe alternative. Why not test yourself by writing down everything you eat, touch or smell. From these notes it is often relatively easy to find out which food item or other factor is most likely to be at the root of your allergic reaction. It is also interesting to see that most people who suffer from allergies also appear to be lacking in calcium. Research by Dr Vogel on the calcium supplement Urticalcin showed that when it was prescribed to an allergic person together with kelp and *Harpagophytum* many of the allergic reactions seemed to diminish or disappear altogether. The highly regarded Dr Len Mervyn, a frequent co-lecturer of mine, has studied in depth all aspects of calcium, and he has developed a new calcium citrate which is easily digested by the body. This development has proved particularly useful to people who are allergic.

Another problem constantly encountered with asthmatic conditions is the accompanying allergy to food additives. Some people seem to develop an allergic reaction to food which contains certain chemical additives or preservatives and it is important that the asthmatic or bronchitic patient checks all food labels to see which additives it contains. The most common additives are tartrazine, the preservatives sulphur dioxide and benzoic acid and the antioxidant BHT. Asthma in one form or another, or skin rashes, are often caused by these particular additives. It has been claimed that at least one person in every hundred is allergic to tartrazine and as this is widely used in many snack foods, it may well be one of the worst offenders as far as allergies go. The same statistical information is relevant to sulphur dioxide, which is also present in many foods and drinks, vegetable spreads and pickles and bear in mind that allergic reactions ascribed to food colourings and additives are now very common indeed. Make a habit of studying the food labels when shopping, as it is not advisable to consume synthetic foods containing many chemicals. Much more investigation is needed into the severe allergic reactions that attack the body's defence system. I do not doubt that a large percentage of all cases of allergies, skin rashes, sinus problems, hay fever and asthma, can be traced back to many of the supposedly harmless food additives.

It is often very sad when there is an allergy to pets. This frequently presents us with a painful dilemma when we have to decide whether or not to part with our four-legged friends — as friends indeed they are. Do not, however, make your decision too hastily. If you suspect that you are allergic to your animal friend, first of all check the symptoms. If you experience itchiness or red eyes, an unusual nasal discharge, shortage of breath, coughing spells followed by wheezing, a blocked nose, or a tendency to rub the eyes and/or nose frequently, then these could well be caused by an allergy to pets. When the immune system is considerably weakened or under severe attack, this could invite stronger allergic reactions. Try using a homoeopathic antidote; alternatively in phytotherapy we also have numerous remedies that are most effective for allergic reactions. I count myself fortunate that I have been able to help so many of my patients to identify and treat their allergies thanks to some of these wonderful natural remedies.

Remember that if you have even a slight allergy to pets, you must ensure that the pet is always kept out of the bedroom. General advice to all allergy sufferers is to keep everything as dust-free as possible. Sometimes when vacuuming or dusting it may pay to wear a mask. Make sure that there are some air purifiers in the house and watch woollen, cotton and nylon materials, which can easily retain pets' hairs.

Many allergic patients can be hypersensitive to perfumes, including those in after-shaves, bath oils and foams, shampoos and washing powders, to name but a few possibilities. Often it is better to use a foam mattress and to do away with feather pillows or continental quilts. Bedding should be of 100 per cent cotton or cotton flannel, and special non-allergic pillows are commercially available for just such purposes. Do not leave magazines or newspapers lying around in the bedroom; nor is the bedroom a suitable place for plants or flowers. Keep your bedroom as clean as possible to avoid any unnecessary risks. Allow absolutely no smoking in the bedroom. These factors are all very important, as well as careful dietary management, which I have already mentioned.

It may be helpful to use cod liver oil, oil of evening primrose, or vitamin B, which all have anti-allergic properties. One of the finest remedies, which has been especially designed for this purpose is called Immuno-strength. This combination remedy contains, among other ingredients, *Echinacea purpurea* and devil's claw — both outstanding herbs — and a range of vitamins, minerals and trace elements. The herbs contained in Immuno-strength have been used for hundreds of years to support the natural defence efforts of the body. The vitamins and minerals it contains are important for the correct functioning of the immune system. Immuno-strength also contains an unusual ingredient — thymus gland concentrate. The T-cells of the immune system mature in the thymus and it is a key immune system organ. This remedy is marketed by Nature's Best, and over the years it has proved to be very successful, particularly when taken in combination with some of the other remedies mentioned earlier. The diet should contain lots of fresh fruit and vegetables, honey, onions, leeks, garlic, vitamins A and C, and herbal teas.

If there is a suspicion that a food allergy is causing asthmatic bronchitis or a related condition, it may be wise to follow the simple measures of elimination to ascertain the most likely allergens. For this purpose I have designed an elimination diet, which we also refer to as the *Stone Age Diet*. It is suitable for children as well as adults and before proceeding to a more elaborate exclusion diet, I suggest that this diet is followed for a period of four weeks. The instructions are given below.

The "Stone Age Diet"
Before beginning:
1. Keep a record of all symptoms for one week before starting the diet.

2. Decide and purchase the foods that will be required.
3. Follow the diet to the letter.

Avoid all the following:

Milk	Chocolate, ice-cream and sweets
Wheat and other cereals	All food colourings
Eggs	All additives
Corn	Tobacco
Sugar	All medication
Citrus fruits	(discuss with doctor beforehand)

Foods that may be eaten:

Meat — meat, fish and poultry (but no pork products).
Vegetables — (except corn); all salads; nuts (except peanuts).
All fruit — except citrus fruits.
Sweeteners — may use a little honey or maple syrup.
Drinks — Malvern water, unsweetened grape juice, apple juice, pineapple juice (natural, not carbonated, not sweetened), herbal teas.
Cooking oil — use sunflower or safflower oil.

Follow this diet for four weeks and keep a daily record of all symptoms. It will often be possible by doing this to identify the nutrients that are offensive to your system.

If by this elimination process you have still not been able to pinpoint the particular allergen, then I would advise that the food allergy elimination diet is followed, as mentioned on page 87 of my book *Viruses, Allergies and the Immune System*. Alternatively, this is another test that can be used to discover allergies, known as the "Pulse Test".

Discovering an allergy using the "Pulse Test"
Begin by recording carefully everything you eat at every

meal for about a week. In addition, take your pulse at the following times each day during the week:

—before rising (in a lying down position before you get out of bed in the morning);

—just before each meal;

—three times (at thirty-minute intervals) after each meal;

—just before going to bed.

This is a total of fourteen pulse counts each day.

How to take your pulse

The most convenient spot is at the wrist, an inch and a half below the base of the thumb and three-quarters of an inch from the end of the wrist. Place the first two fingers of the right hand on the left wrist so that they cover this spot. When counting your pulse have a watch or clock with a second hand close in view. Pick up the pulse with the fingertips and wait until the second hand reaches sixty. Then count on the next pulse beat and continue counting the beats until the second hand has made a complete circuit and returned to sixty, which will make the completion of one minute. The number of the pulse beats counted in one minute is the pulse rate.

Always either sit or stand when taking the pulse. Be consistent throughout. If the highest pulse count that you get every day for a week is not over 85 and if it is the same each day, you are probably not allergic to any food. On any given day the range from the lowest count to the highest count will probably not be more than sixteen beats.

A count greater than 85 points to a food allergy.

If the highest count varies more than two beats from day to day, you are certainly allergic; that is, if on Monday

81

you have a count of 72, on Tuesday 78, Wednesday 76, Thursday 71.

If your pulse rates seem to indicate that you are not allergic to any food you ate on a particular day, but on the other days the jump from high to low is great or there is a count above 85, then it is wise to eat for several days the same food that you had on the non-allergic day, adding to it only one food at a time, to see if you can locate the offending food.

Do not smoke
Smoking complicates the whole picture. There are many people who are not allergic to any food but who are allergic to tobacco. Patients *must* give up smoking while they are doing the test.

Finding your specific allergen(s)
You may discover that you are allergic to something you eat every day, but you do not know specifically what it is. This is how you can isolate the specific irritant in question.

Find a free weekend when your time is your own and you can experiment to your heart's content. Eat nothing for dinner on the Friday night. The following morning, begin your test by eating one ordinary kind of food at a time and taking your pulse just before eating and at half-hour intervals after eating this *single* food. You might first eat a slice of bread. Next you might take a boiled egg. Do the three pulse tests at half-hour intervals after eating, then try another food — and so on. In this way you can test ten or twelve single foods over the course of a weekend. It does not matter how much of the single food you eat, providing you do not mix it with any other food.

During the course of your pulse testing do not decide to take up long-distance running or anything equally strenuous and demanding. Any exertion to which you are not accustomed can easily raise your pulse. Carefully note your results together with the records of your pulse beat and take these to your practitioner at your next consultation.

If approached in the correct way, allergies can be overcome. Expensive tests or treatment are rarely necessary and much misery can be avoided. I will conclude this chapter with an article from the *Sunday Correspondent* of 22 October 1989, which contains some interesting facts and figures.

No rash promises
Thirty years ago asthma was unknown on Tristan da Cunha, the tiny British island in the windswept south Atlantic. Today it is afflicting the hardy inhabitants in increasing numbers. The same illness began laying low the tribespeople of Papua New Guinea only in the 1970s. In Japan, cedar pollen allergy — the Japanese equivalent of hay fever — was unknown before 1963. Now it is claiming thousands of new victims every year.

In Britain and all around the world, allergies are on the increase. The trends for all the major conditions — hay fever, asthma and eczema — are the same: steeply upwards. It is as if the human immune system, deprived of a decent infection or two to fight in the modern, sterile world, is turning in on itself for a bit of self-destructive mayhem.

In many developing countries, asthma is unknown in rural villages but common in the cleaner, modern cities. The immune systems of those who live in the primitive villages are fully engaged fending off the daily assault from parasites and other biological invaders. But when they move to the cleaner city, their immune systems search relentlessly for new enemies to overthrow — such as the microscopic creatures found in house dust. When the body takes a biochemical sledgehammer to crack a mite — in this case the house dust mite — you have asthma.

This seems to be what happened in Papua New Guinea. During the 1970s, the Australian government sent boatloads of blankets to Papua New Guinea by way of aid. The tribespeople took to them eagerly, wearing them by day and sleeping under them by night. Since house dust mites feed on the tiny particles of skin continually sloughed off our bodies, the Papua New Guinea variety had a feast — and the tribespeople were soon wheezing hard.

In Britain, our version of the Papua New Guinea blankets is the warm, humid boxes in which we choose to live, with close-fitting window frames that don't let in draughts and soft furnishings that hold dust. Wall-to-wall carpets mean wall-to-wall house dust mites. Rising living standards, in Torquay as in Tristan da Cunha, mean rising allergies.

Rising pollution levels worldwide are also thought to be sensitising more people to familiar allergic substances like pollen. In Japan, the rise in hay fever (cedar pollen allergy) has been linked to the rise in car ownership, especially of the diesel-powered kind. One influential study showed that mice immunised with diesel particles acquired allergies to a range of other substances. But the pollution theory cuts little ice in Tristan da Cunha.

There are other puzzles. Was Japanese hay fever unknown or merely unrecognised before 1963? It is impossible to prove either way. We are better at detecting allergies today and readier to suspect them as the cause of certain symptoms. So how real is the rise?

The children of mothers who smoked during pregnancy are more likely to develop allergies — and smoking among women has increased steadily since the Second World War. Could this explain our growing sensitivity? But eczema, suffered chiefly by children, has seen one of the most consistent increases and it is *not* linked to smoking among mothers. Smokers themselves are more likely to suffer allergic reactions to many substances — lending weight to the pollution theory — but *less* likely to react to some, like chemicals.

The role of the mind in allergy is the subject of further confusion. Increased publicity about allergy has undoubtedly led more people to suspect they have one. A survey of 20,000 people in 1988 found that one in twelve believed they were sensitive to food additives. But when they took part in a blind tasting of foods with a range of additives, fewer than one in 1,000 showed a response. Many of these people had a genuine reaction when they knew what they were eating, indicating that anxiety plays an important part in producing or augmenting the response.

But the leap from this finding to dismissing allergy as all in the mind is not only false but dangerous. An "immune system malfunction", as the doctors insist on calling it, can be life-threatening. As asthma has risen sharply in Britain, so have the number of deaths, now hitting 2,000 a year. Most of them could be avoided with proper treatment delivered in time.

However, the incidence of the disease is increasing faster than our capacity to educate people about its potentially lethal consequences. Even among doctors there is a lingering belief that the cause is psychological and the cure a lecture of the "pull your socks up" variety. Hence the campaign by the Asthma Society, which aims to encourage potential sufferers to go for a check-up.

For one development, sufferers may be grateful: allergy is at last professionally respectable. Though still starved of funds, research is delivering new hope. Recent findings have suggested a high-salt diet may aggravate asthma. Trials are being carried out with acaricides, a kind of insect spray that slaughters house dust mites, which has had "encouraging" results in Australia, where it was developed.

Research by Tak Lee, Professor of Allergy at Guy's Hospital, London, has shown that fish oil supplements in the diet can prevent asthmatic attacks in the laboratory. Trials are soon to take place to see whether the same effect can be achieved outside the laboratory.

But investigation of the hereditary basis of allergy holds out the greatest promise. Allergies run in families. A team at Churchill Hospital, Oxford, has reported in the *Lancet* that they had traced the allergy gene to chromosome 11. "This is where the answer is going to lie," said Professor Lee. "If we can identify the genes then we can think about a cure."

8

Hay Fever

IT IS ALMOST unbelievable but is sadly an established fact that in Britain alone there are ten million hay fever sufferers. For some, the only symptoms may be no more than a runny nose or itchy eyes, but desperate sufferers will go to great lengths and be prepared to spend a small fortune on any treatment that will give them a measure of relief. Of course, the nature of the treatment depends on the severity of the allergy. Some people may find a nasal spray to be effective whereas others may prefer an injection or course of injections; others still seem to find relief in more aggressive cures. And yet, I can assure you that in the field of allergies alternative medicine has more to offer than conventional medicine.

As summer approaches most of us look forward to the long hours of daylight and to long evenings spent enjoying the late sunshine in the garden, but those who are subjected to a pollen allergy await summer with mixed feelings. They know that an allergic reaction may well lead to attacks that are akin to asthma symptoms. There will be much sneezing as well as runny noses, caused by blockage of the Eustachian tubes connecting the ears and throat. Those people will often go to any lengths to forestall or avoid these conditions.

Hay fever affects not only the tissues of the nose, throat and eyes, it also affects the immune system, severely irritates the nose, and causes great suffering. Statistics suggest that there is a real danger that one in three hay fever sufferers will become asthmatic. With children especially, complications are sometimes experienced: light asthmatic or hay fever symptoms can easily trigger an outbreak of allergic eczema and the child could become emotional and nervous. Sometimes it is difficult to isolate the cause of hay fever, as the allergy may only be to a specific kind of pollen. Depending on the time of year, the reactions that occur will enable the practitioner to pinpoint the cause more accurately.

Little is known about the function of the eosinophil cells. We do know that sensitivity to pollen expresses itself in an attack on these cells through the mucus contained in the nose. These eosinophil cells usually show up in the blood tests of allergic asthma sufferers, thus confirming the diagnosis. Reactions to the pollen of certain trees, especially oak and birch, and to grass pollen, are certainly well known. But it is also possible for fungi to act as an allergen. In most cases desensitising is of prime importance, and once the correct diagnosis has been established hay fever patients can take action at the beginning of the season, usually around April, by building up their immunity to the offensive factors. Remember that antibiotics, antihistamines or cortico-steroid treatments are rarely necessary, for there are plenty of natural remedies ideally suited to overcoming these problems.

It is sometimes claimed that hay fever may be hereditary because the sufferer's parents or grandparents are known to have experienced such problems. I don't believe that this is altogether true. Indeed, hay fever can affect anyone who possesses an allergic tendency or oversensitivity. Hay fever sufferers can do much to help themselves by modifying their diet as it is believed that the allergens are composed protein molecules, which are larger than the normal proteins when absorbed in the blood. For years I have told patients that the real causes of hay fever are hidden in the immune system. It is our individual defensive response to an invasion of pollen that will affect the sensitive immune system, and an imbalance may result. For this reason it is essential that hay fever sufferers carefully reconsider their dietary regime, as chemical additives and preservatives and a high protein diet may exacerbate the problem.

One particular contributory factor that is often over-looked is the possibility that because of some dietary imbalance the liver is not receiving the nourishment it requires. Moreover, any extreme emotions or traumas will affect the immune defence system, sometimes causing metabolic disorders and/or hypersensitivity. These factors may lead to overstimulation, followed by allergic reactions and in the worst possible situation causing a case of ultra-intoxification. Detoxification will thus be essential and this can be done by following the dietary guidelines provided in Chapter 7. Be especially sparing with animal protein and salt, while at the same time introducing plenty of honey and fruit into the diet. Try this regime for a few days if you wish. Starchy, sugary food should be reduced to the bare minimum and, as has been said before, no dairy produce whatsoever is allowed.

Clearing any congestion is of great importance and in this respect the early naturopaths had a point when they advised patients to take plenty of Epsom salts baths. Epsom salts are not expensive, and it would be worth your while immersing yourself fully in a bath filled with nice hot water to which has been added a handful of Epsom salts. Remain in the bath for 10–15 minutes then retire to a warm bed with a hot water bottle. Every night and morning sniff some ice-cold water with a few drops of lemon juice added; this too will relieve your catarrh. Splashing the face with cold water is also beneficial.

I expect that the average hay fever sufferer will already be aware that alcohol, nicotine, chocolate and spices should be avoided. Instead of coffee or tea, try drinking a herbal tea or a lemon and honey drink, which are much more sensible and will help to alleviate the allergic condition.

Medically, there are a number of ways to treat hay fever. On average, homoeopathic treatment should be started no later than February, and this can take the form of injections of formic acid. The use of *Kalium iod.* D4 and *Arsenicum album* D4 is also recommended for hay fever. However, in my experience one of the best remedies is Pollinosan. This is an exceptional hay fever remedy and I have seen proof of its success all over the world. The results of research undertaken in eight general practices in the Netherlands showed that 75 per cent of the hay fever patients had benefited greatly from Pollinosan. A spokesperson for the research team commented that the general feedback was that the allergic reactions were reduced as soon as Pollinosan was taken and the patients were extremely enthusiastic about this remedy. The tests took place during 1988 and 1989 and a total of 199 patients participated. Of these, 88.5 per cent reported some improvement after using Pollinosan, while 56.8 per cent claimed to be either fully or nearly free of allergic symptoms. Most of these patients had been diagnosed as being allergic to pollen, although it was concluded that even people who suffered from another form of inhalation allergy, for example to house mites or pets, also reported great improvement. No less than 76.9 per cent of the patients who suffered from hay fever as well as house mite allergies experienced a reasonable to very considerable improvement.

Pollinosan contains the following ingredients:

—*Ammi visnaga*, which is a powerful antispasmodic useful in the treatment of asthma, whooping cough and hay fever;

—*Aralia racemosa*, renowned for its expectorant and diuretic characteristics;

—*Cardiospermum halicacabum*, an expectorant and antispasmodic and a very useful ingredient for any allergic problems;

—*Larrea mexicana*, used for coughs and colds and possessing an anti-microbiotic action;

—*Luffa perculata*, which has long been used to treat nasal catarrh and sinus infections in ancient Colombian folk medicine;

—*Okoubaka aubrevillei*, used to treat nasal complaints and headaches;

—*Thryalis glauca*, used in the treatment of allergies which cause hay fever, asthmatic bronchitis, rhinitis and other allergic skin problems.

It is advised that patients continue taking this remedy until the problems have cleared up completely. No contra-indications have ever been reported with this remedy and it must be considered as a major breakthrough in the treatment of hay fever.

For the minority of people who have the misfortune of failing to respond to the use of Pollinosan, I generally advise that they use *Galeopsis* and *Harpagophytum*. Herbal teas, sweetened with honey, can also help, particularly the following, which may be taken singly or in combinations: thyme, marjoram, hyssop, lavender and stinging nettle. Compresses of witch hazel and chamomile often provide relief during severe attacks. The same is true of tissue salts and specifically I would recommend *Nat. mur.*, especially to soothe any itching, while *Nat. phos.* will relax any spasms. Make sure that your intake of vitamins, minerals and trace elements is adequate, remembering that under the circumstances the vitamin B complex, manganese, chromium and iron are the most required.

Several times already I have stressed the benefits of honey; it is at its best when taken straight from the honeycomb. Royal jelly is also a richly concentrated nutrient that will help to strengthen the immune system. Another remedy that is gaining wider recognition for its health-giving characteristics is propolis, which is especially useful when suffering from colds and influenza. A recent discovery is the ioniser. Many patients have asked me for my opinion of this device and my reaction is enthusiastic. I am certain that hay fever sufferers will be pleased by the relief obtained from an ioniser. Aromatherapy also has a lot to offer, and last summer one of my patients claimed that acupuncture had been the only treatment that had been effective in his battle against hay fever. He told me that after only one session of acupuncture the mucous discharge and the sinus congestion had almost cleared, as had the allergic symptoms. So, acupuncture, that centuries-old Chinese treatment, still manages to surprise us in unexpected ways.

A new remedy to which many of my patients have responded very well is ImuGuard, which is a concentrated version of whey, the watery part of cow's milk that has been recommended since the time of Hippocrates.

More specifically, ImuGuard is based on AIC, or active immunoglobin concentrate. Immunoglobins are proteins with a specific antibody action against antigens, the many substances that are able to provoke a response from the immune system. The protein, fat and water mixture of dairy whey is the part of milk that contains the immunoglobins, enzymes and a specific set of immune system proteins known as complement that help keep the gastro-intestinal tract of suckling calves healthy. Similarly, the human immune system takes some time to mature, and during this period the human infant benefits from the passive protection passed from the mother through her breast milk. Researchers believe they have unlocked the secret of whey, and that the active antibodies and enzymes present in AIC explain why it has been valued as a food for so long. Although no studies of AIC have been carried out on humans, it is known that our intestines contain large populations of parasites and a mixture of friendly and unfriendly micro-organisms. The immune system manufactures antibodies whose role it is to neutralise the unfriendly residents and so maintain the balance in favour of the friendly ones.

With persistent cases of hay fever, the remedy ImuGuard has proved highly successful together with Pure-Gar, a garlic-based remedy. Both remedies are marketed by Nature's Best and the latter is claimed to be very much closer to the nutritional profile of natural, raw garlic than other garlic supplements. Without a doubt, garlic has an anti-toxic effect and is a marvellous natural antibiotic.

If the advice given in this chapter is heeded, hay fever patients can be hopeful of enjoying themselves next summer and participating in any sports activities in the open air without experiencing the usual problems of hay fever.

9

Sinusitis and Rhinitis

SINUSITIS IS AN inflammation of the accessory nasal sinuses — and this is a much larger problem than is generally recognised. I have often been consulted by patients who were in despair, not knowing where to turn for relief from the pain and discomfort. Unless we have suffered from this condition it is difficult to comprehend what a sinus sufferer has to put up with or how chronic this type of condition can be. The sinus patient can be affected by inadequate drainage or the projecting growths of mucous membrane inside the nose, also known as polyps.

In the case of chronic sinusitis — inflammation of the mucous membranes in the nose — we must be aware that this problem could eventually develop into a more serious health condition. It has been known for the problem to develop as a result of allergic reactions or dental irregularities. Unfortunately, I have had to treat many patients who were suffering from such problems and complaining about dreadful headaches, nasal discharge, dizziness and aches and pains elsewhere. Sometimes the symptoms will be localised, but it is not unusual for them to spread to other areas and develop into a variety of pains not immediately associated with sinusitis, until we question the patient carefully. It is also possible for the patient to run a temperature and feel feverish. If the problem is allowed to become chronic, the symptoms may travel from the forehead to the cheeks and sometimes through the whole of the head.

Finding the cause of a sinus condition may not be as straightforward as we would like, because it can be due to a combination of many things. X-rays and nasal examinations can point us in the right direction. An average case of sinusitis can be treated with one of a number of drugs. Painkillers may provide relief, but only temporarily as they will not treat the cause of the problem. Over the years I have come to the conclusion that nine times out of ten when a chronic sinusitis condition has been allowed to develop, it has resulted from an allergy. Occasionally I have found the cause to be a minor displacement, which can often be corrected with osteopathy. Usually the patient will have to be re-educated with regard to blowing the nose. This should always be done with the mouth open and one nostril only should be blown at a time.

There is no doubt that people who suffer from sinusitis, especially if the condition has become chronic, need help. It is not necessarily an easy condition to cure, as it can be extremely persistent and uncomfortable. Help is available, however; alternative medicine has various methods which offer not only relief, but often a cure. First and foremost the sinusitis and chronic rhinitis patient would be wise to go through a dietary elimination process to discover the most likely offending factor that is causing the allergy. This can then be dealt with. To simplify this process, I can tell you that in the majority of cases I have come across, the cause was found to be one or more dairy products. As I have said before, these allergies are more common than one might think, and where they have been identified, goat's milk or soya milk can be used instead. The dietary guidelines I have already provided for asthmatic patients are applicable to sinusitis patients too, remembering in particular to increase the use of honey and to reduce the intake of salt, spices, alcohol and coffee. Introduce oats and fruit and vegetable juices to the diet, especially carrot, blackcurrant, lemon and orange juice. Remember to use garlic wherever possible because of its wonderful antibacterial properties.

An element of fashion seems to creep into everything nowadays, but this has long been the case with medicine. In this respect a number of periods can be very clearly identified. Centuries ago bloodletting and enemas were very much in fashion; more recently we have gone through a period where antibiotics or cortisone treatment were considered the panacea. For a while tonsils and adenoids were removed without a second thought for little or no reason at all.

Shortly after the Second World War I had my tonsils removed, although my parents were not in favour, but then it was the done thing. Later on in life I have regretted this, because unless the tonsils are very inflamed or infected, there is no reason for this operation. Even if the tonsils are swollen to such an extent that there appears to be no other course of action, homoeopathy and phytotherapy have remedies that will help shrink them, and which can benefit them in other ways, as well as eliminating infections. However, I was a victim of the prevailing fashion and now when I have a cold my sinuses are easily affected. It should be remembered that the removal of the tonsils and adenoids has a great bearing on the development of certain diseases.

People who are affected by sinusitis, rhinitis or related asthmatic problems should never smoke and could even be affected by smoky surroundings. Recently I came across some startling figures: it seems that in 1933 an estimated 14,000,000,000 cigarettes were smoked annually by the female population alone in Britain. I doubt if that figure is still so frighteningly high, yet many people still do not seem to realise that nicotine is a deadly poison and that even one drop, if taken undiluted, could kill a person. Why should we dope ourselves with nicotine, alcohol or other addictive drugs, when so much more happiness can be obtained by living closer to nature?

Naturopathy offers a number of sensible and effective approaches to treating sinusitis and rhinitis problems. One of the lesser known methods is hydrotherapy. In my book *Water — Healer or Poison?* I have given quite a few suggestions for this purpose and one of these is as follows: soak a piece of towel in hot water to which some chamomile has been added, wring it out and place it over the painful area for 2–3 minutes. Repeat this procedure three or four times. Then follow this by placing ice-cold compresses over the same area.

You may laugh at my next suggestion, but if you are experiencing a lot of pain in a localised area, try bandaging a fresh cabbage leaf over the exact location. Almost immediately the acute throbbing pain will diminish. Many people are derisory about this old-fashioned treatment until they eventually try it themselves. Sometimes patients decide that this is just an old wives' tale and that it is too much work and instead they prefer to wash out the sinuses. However, especially in cases of chronic sinusitis, the effects of a sinus wash will only be temporary. Some of the old-fashioned treatments may be of more use than is initially apparent and to obtain effective relief it is definitely worthwhile trying some alternative medicine.

Two homoeopathic remedies, namely *Hepar sulph.* and *Cinnabaris* are often used in the treatment of sinusitis and rhinitis. The latter is ideally suited for the treatment of frontal sinusitis and sinusitis around the upper jaw with suppuration. For ear infections and sub-acute and chronic inflammation of the sinus passages near the nose, or the mucous membranes in the nose, it is also beneficial. *Hepar sulph.* is also used to bring infections to a head; for coughs, croupy coughs, bronchitis, inflammatory colds, sinusitis and inflammation of the ear and middle ear, it is an excellent remedy. Both *Hepar sulph.* and *Cinnabaris* are prescribed in homoeopathic combinations which also contain *Mag. phos.* and *Kal. chlor.* Rubbing some Poho oil onto the affected areas is also recommended and if the sinusitis problem is chronic, Usneasan should be taken. Don't forget about the well-proven remedies cod liver oil, propolis and B-Pollen. Inhalations of lemon, eucalyptus and Poho oil are also highly recommended. Finally, to help the immune system you can use a preparation like Immuno-strength, or vitamin A, betacarotene, vitamin C, vitamin E and if necessary some vitamin B.

On the subject of rhinitis I would again like to point out that there are different kinds of this condition, namely allergic rhinitis, chronic rhinitis and atrophic rhinitis. These are all nasal disturbances either with acute inflammation and hypersensitivity or a chronic inflammatory process with thickening of the nasal mucosa. In atrophic rhinitis there is also crust formation, which could make the condition more severe. This, of course, is an extreme form of nasal catarrh, and can prove very difficult to treat.

In the case of chronic rhinitis it would be wise to follow a fasting regime followed by a change in diet. A low-protein diet, avoiding all dairy produce, is needed. In all cases of rhinitis one could use, apart from the homoeopathic remedies *Hepar sulph.* and *Cinnabaris*, Dr Vogel's remedy Petaforce. For inhalations use menthol, Olbas oil, chamomile, eucalyptus, lavender, pine or thyme, all of which will prove helpful. Immuno-strength, together with a vitamin A supplement is also recommended. In serious cases vitamin A is required by the thymus gland, the key organ of the immune system; the mucous membranes of the lungs, nose, throat and mouth also depend on it. In fact, a supplementary dose of vitamin A will aid all the organs of the body.

To summarise, then, various types of sinusitis and rhinitis can be helped by adopting a revised dietary approach in conjunction with homoeopathic and herbal treatment, vitamin supplements and inhalations.

10

Influenza

MY REASON FOR including influenza in a book on asthma and bronchitis is that it is more than likely to have been the initial cause of the conditions dealt with elsewhere in this book. In many cases, asthma, pneumonia, bronchitis and other related problems appear to have taken hold as the result of a bout of influenza. I have been told many times by patients, when they were relating their case history, that they were fine until they were hit by a flu bug. We dismiss this illness so easily as "only a bout of flu" or "only a bug"; we fully expect to be back on our feet in a few days' time at the most. Let's not forget that influenza is a highly contagious and acute disease caused by a virus. This virus will cause a fever, aches and pains and an inflammation of the respiratory mucous membranes. So, it doesn't pay to under-estimate the effects of influenza. Granted, in cases of acute influenza there is usually a speedy recovery. Nevertheless, the patient will have had a raised temperature and to make a speedy recovery, rest, some sensible remedies and good care are essential. I still believe that in any case of influenza, when the patient has a raised temperature, rest is essential. A number of remedies can be used to overcome this condition completely.

I always have had great regard for my grandmother's medical knowledge. She was an excellent practitioner and advised many patients to eat beetroot or to drink a few glasses of beetroot or carrot juice for even a minor attack of flu. It may be an old-fashioned remedy, but I assure you that it assists the patient's recovery.

Consider some of our loosely termed "twentieth-century diseases" and I promise you that many can be traced back to a possible viral attack that was initially caused by influenza. Had this first complaint been treated with consideration, it is unlikely that it would have developed into a more serious condition. Following a bout of influenza, bacterial pneumonia could result due to a haemolytic streptococcus, staphylcococcus or a pneumococcus. These bacteria can be fatal. In 1918 ten million people died from what was considered "only a bout of flu".

Myalgic encephalomyelitis (ME), also known as "yuppy flu", is still very much a mystery. Of the hundreds of ME patients I have treated nearly all had suffered from glandular fever.

Glandular fever is an acute infectious disease. It is often classified as a lymph adenopathy, and the lymphatic tissue is usually involved. When treating glandular fever it is essential that the remedies are selected carefully so as to ensure the complete recovery of the lymphatic system. Although we know that glandular fever is an infectious disease, we still have insufficient knowledge of how exactly the body is affected by it and thus how best to effect a cure or, better still, how to

101

avoid falling prey to this illness in the first place. During the course of my years of practice, I have learned, however, that the treatment of glandular fever must be tackled seriously, as in many cases the illness has provided the background for the development of some of these "twentieth-century diseases". The throat, glands or liver are often infiltrated by lymphocytes, and by taking this into consideration during the treatment of glandular fever we may save patients from many further illnesses. In the next chapter, which looks at throat conditions, I will deal with this aspect in greater detail.

During the course of an attack of influenza the body's temperature can rise to 101°F (38.3°C) or even 103°F (39.4°C) and it is this rise in temperature that is often the most worrying factor. However, I should point out that the body needs to pass through a healing crisis in order to fight and overcome the invaders that have attacked our general health. Suppressing a fever serves to weaken the immune system, so that it may not be able to rise to the challenge and fight off the invaders when attacked on a future occasion.

A persistent fever can be frightening and instead of seeking a total recovery, we often set out to suppress the coughs and pains that are merely symptoms. To this end we try to control a secondary bacterial invasion by chemical means, not realising that by doing so we might be laying ourselves wide open to future problems such as bronchial sinusitis or pneumonia. With good understanding and the correct treatment methods this need not be necessary. This is the reason for my insistence that influenza should be taken seriously and not just shrugged off as an unfortunate annual nuisance.

Much research has taken place in an effort to gain more insight into the influenza germ. In naturopathy we believe that it is not so much the germ as the condition of the individual's general health that matters. An impaired immune system and a high level of toxicity are like an open invitation to invading germs. It is interesting that people who live according to their naturopathic principles seldom suffer from flu or a cold. The picture is rather different for people who pay little attention to their diet and who sit in stuffy rooms and spend inordinate amounts of time in front of the television screen. The more oxygen and energy are produced, the better chance we have of resisting infection. Flu epidemics usually take place during or after the winter, when our natural reserves are bound to be a little below par. Individually, we generally find that it is after times of stress or over-eating that we have less resistance to colds or infections. Influenza, according to naturopathic understanding, can be regarded as a self-cleansing procedure. The body is undertaking to rid itself of toxic and alien material, which it considers did not belong there in the first place. This again underlines the importance of my insistence that influenza be treated carefully, because if it were to be suppressed, or treated with unsuitable drugs, kidney, liver or heart problems could result. All the research still being undertaken on influenza would be unnecessary if patients were only prepared to follow the sensible naturopathic rules and methods and so avoid more serious and persistent after-effects.

While the fever rages a fasting programme should be followed. As long as the patient drinks plenty of fluids, the fever will eventually begin to abate. An all fruit and/or liquid diet is advised. By following such a diet the body will eliminate much toxic matter and a thorough cleaning will be achieved.

In recent years we have increasingly heard of people who suffer from flu on an annual basis. This is absolutely unnecessary, and should this be the case, I can recommend Detox Box Programme (Dr Vogel's). This is one of the best cleansing programmes I know for detoxifying the whole body and strengthening the immune system.

The programme consists of a combination of five remedies, and is better known as the Rasayana course. The remedies are as follows:

1. Nephrosolid, an excellent kidney and bladder cleanser;
2. Rasayana 1, a herbal laxative and blood cleanser;
3. Rasayana 2, stimulates the production of bile and cleanses the blood;
4. Echinaforce, stimulates the immune system;
5. Goldengrass tea, better known as kidney tea, which stimulates kidney function.

The Rasayana course is thus a blood-cleansing, regulating, and detoxifying programme; it promotes the digestion, the secretion of bile and the discharge of urine, stimulates intestinal and glandular activity and eliminates poisonous substances. Together with Echinaforce, the Rasayana course provides us with a safe way to rid the body of toxic material and waste matter.

Remember, fever is not a disease, more a symptom of disease. It is one of those wonderful alarm bells in the body that tells us that there is something wrong. Listen to your body and you will learn to recognise when there may be something amiss. Of course, this observation is not limited to influenza; all symptoms should be carefully treated, as different signals may be an early indication of approaching dysfunctions.

A famous physician once said: "Give me the power to induce a fever and I will cure all disease." This is a momentous statement, but to my mind it contains tremendous wisdom which should not be ignored. Let me give you a few practical hints in cases of fever. Fever may be caused by a high level of intoxication and appropriate action will therefore be required. This could take the form of an enema made from an infusion of herbs. To reduce a fever I would suggest that a combination of chickweed and bayberry bark is used, together with the echinacea flower. Drinking rosehip tea will also be helpful. Cider vinegar compresses on the calves of the legs and on the back have proved effective. For children with a fever, the homoeopathic remedies *Ferr. phos.* 12x, *Aconitum* 4x and *Belladonna* can be useful. With children and old people, it is essential that they have plenty of rest and are kept warm. Vitamin C and the herbal remedy Influaforce has been used by a German general practitioner in the treatment of thousands of patients for flu with a success rate of 99 per cent. This particular doctor prescribes natural remedies, especially for people who have a low resistance. He advocates the use of *Eupatorium* and claims to have followed up the results of 6,000 patients who had suffered viral attacks and found that 5,922 of these, that is 98.7 per cent, reacted very well indeed. The North American Indians used to use *Eupatorium* to treat "flu-like" cases and in particular as a treatment for forest fever. *Eupatorium* can also be used in a complex remedy and is especially recommended for secondary infections such as throat or tonsil infections during or after influenza.

I would now like to add a few further notes regarding the dietary approach required during an attack of influenza. Under these conditions the digestive system is especially sluggish and the absorption of food will be much more difficult. It is advisable, therefore, to avoid eggs, fish, meat and cheese, all of which will be found difficult to digest. Instead, take more fruit juices. Remember to select fruit juices that are low in acid, so grape or blackcurrant juice would be an excellent choice. As always honey is beneficial and when the digestive system has recovered sufficiently garlic or garlic capsules can be reintroduced. To get the digestive system completely back in order, you could use the excellent Obbekjaer peppermint remedy, either in powder or tablet form. Porridge oats are excellent for strengthening the nervous system. Throughout my medical practice I have stressed the benefits to be obtained by starting the day with a breakfast of oats — *Avena sativa*. Oats not only strengthen the nervous system, but they are also excellent for keeping the cholesterol level down. Moreover, they are highly effective for catarrh and colds, and will even help soothe an inflammation of the stomach and intestines.

Prevention is always better than cure and the stronger we arm ourselves against flu or colds the more we will benefit. When our immune system is impaired we will become more susceptible to infections, which in turn may lead to more serious problems. Nutrition is therefore very important, but nowadays we can also choose supplements to achieve better immunity. We live in an age that inundates us with so many potentially harmful toxins. The air we breathe carries pollutants, amongst them sulphur dioxide and a variety of other chemicals. The same can be said about our drinking water. We should also realise that as a result of interference, our food contains additives and colourings, which can cause numerous digestive and absorption problems. Anti-nutrients increase the need for specific nutrients to detoxify the body. Anti-nutrients such as heavy metals, lead, mercury, cadmium, caffeine, tobacco, alcohol, sugar, etc. are hidden dangers. Under the circumstances it makes sense to pay some extra attention to our diet in order to prevent secondary diseases taking hold. If we are practical we will not stop at adopting a well-balanced diet; we will also take some supplements to strengthen our immunity. Vitamin C is one of our best allies in this respect as it is a unique nutrient: it is needed throughout the whole of our body as an anti-oxidant.

Remember, prevention is always better than cure.

11

Throat Conditions

IT IS WITH ADMIRATION that I remember the older generation of doctors who would always ask to look at the tongue and throat of their patients. I know that some medical practitioners still do this today, but the practice is much less common than it was. Gone are the times when this was done as a matter of course. This is unfortunate, because the tongue and the throat are excellent indicators of problems elsewhere in the body. In China, where I studied for a while, great store is set on tongue diagnosis, and as a result I often ask my patients if I can see their tongues. Sometimes it is possible to discern a whole case history from the tongue, and at the same time the throat often gives us an indication of present or imminent problems. Throat conditions are often neglected, and it is here that the first indications of problems may be recognised. Unfortunately, people pay little or no attention to such early warning signs and a throat irritation that persists for more than a few days only is usually considered merely as a nuisance.

I was greatly in awe of one of the earliest acupuncture practitioners in Scotland. Although he was an orthodox doctor, he practised acupuncture in a way that commanded great respect. Some people considered his approach rather unorthodox and somewhat barbaric, but without hurting the patient he would know how and where to look for the cause of a problem. He relied on a little piece of equipment producing high-frequency cold-fire spots, which he sometimes pushed as far as possible into the throat of patients, so activating acupuncture points to relieve the problem. He also used this device to seek out infections. He told me about some of the throat infections he had found in patients with degenerative diseases and how this had helped him to learn more about the patient's condition. In this way he was more likely to discover the cause, rather than by studying the other more obvious symptoms. I had great respect for this practitioner and learned much from him, as I came to understand that with an early diagnosis of the cause, the subsequent development of more serious problems could be prevented.

Not long ago I was consulted by a young female patient who had sought help from various practitioners. Despite this, the development of a degenerative disease had not been discovered, for no other reason than an infection in the lymph glands had been overlooked time and again. From an examination of her tongue I was able to draw the correct conclusions and successfully located both the infection and the source of the problem. This proves that some of the old methods are worth holding on to.

I was once consulted by an asthmatic patient who experienced dreadful throat problems. She coughed so much that she paid little attention to the irritation of her throat, because she thought that the ache was a result of the actual coughing, while in fact it was the other way round. This throat pain had started as a forerunner to a chronic throat infection, and asthma was the unpleasant after-effect. The initial sore throat had not been treated and had been allowed to deteriorate into a much more serious condition. It is not only when the tonsils are red and swollen, or covered in white spots, that an antibiotic or other medicine should be given; it is just as important to treat other problems that this condition could trigger off. I cannot count the times when an apparently simple throat irritation has signalled the start of a rheumatic condition, heart or kidney problems, chronic bronchitis or asthma. The risk is there and the root of the problem should be treated from the beginning. It is not only annoying when the throat is sore, but it can tire the patient and can even result in total loss of voice. Resting the throat will often prove helpful, and it may even be all that is needed to completely clear up the problem without any further help. In general, however, what advice should be followed for the treatment of throat problems?

The tonsils and adenoids are part of the lymphoid tissue and serve as a protection. They are frequently subjected to acute and chronic infections and these infections can be caused by a virus or bacteria, including a cold or flu. Acute tonsillitis is an acute inflammation of the tonsils, caused by the group A haemolytic streptococci. Severe pain in the tonsil area may be experienced, accompanied by an extremely high fever. There can be severe discomfort, pain and swelling, as well as coughing or stiffness of the neck. The tonsils are usually very enlarged and covered with red spots with a whitish-yellow head. For such throat conditions I would immediately prescribe *Lachesis*. We can be thankful to Dr Constantin Hering for the discovery of this remarkable remedy, which has saved many lives. *Lachesis* — snake poison — is mostly considered with trepidation, yet when the blood is toxic, *Lachesis* in homoeopathic form is often the solution. For acute or chronic tonsillitis *Lachesis* is more likely to help where other remedies have failed. As tonsillitis can spread an infection, the tissue salts *Kali. mur.* or *Ferr. phos.* can be used to reduce the swollen glands, as can the remedy Molkosan used as a gargle.

A minor throat irritation is often an early indication of a throat infection. When the tonsils become red and swollen and the throat becomes constricted it is time for action. In olden times naturopathic doctors used to ask the patient if he or she was constipated, and in such cases they would advise that castor oil be taken. This helps to evacuate the bowels, which in turn speeds up the healing of throat problems. It is true that recurrent attacks of tonsillitis or other throat problems are often the result of constipation. After fasting on liquids, when the symptoms are beginning to clear, gradually reintro-duce some solids such as fruits and vegetables. If the tonsils and adenoids are badly swollen, take the remedy *Marum verum*, which is effective whenever difficulty with swallowing and inflammation of the tonsils, adenoids and gums are experienced. Because of these character-istics it is often prescribed for pharyngitis, laryngitis and tonsillitis. Drink herbal teas such as sage or thyme, or use cold compresses made using these two herbs. Ice cubes may help to soothe an inflamed throat; even rubbing a lit-tle garlic into the throat may bring quick relief. The latter remedy is often advised for a quinsy throat, which is an acute suppuration located between the tonsils and the pharynx. Again, it is important to gargle with Molkosan

111

and to take Echinaforce. During double-blind trials a number of patients were given either Echinaforce or a placebo. It became apparent that echinacea was highly effective against viruses and bacteria. It was concluded that hyaluron acid, a gel that protects against bacteria and viruses contained in the body tissue, was assisted by the echinacea.

This brings us to pharyngitis. Acute pharyngitis is an inflammation of the pharynx, and is usually caused by a viral infection. The symptoms of this condition include a burning sensation and dryness, the feeling of a lump in the throat, hoarseness, swelling and a red mucus. Acute pharyngitis should be treated without delay, following the guidelines given for tonsillitis, so as to prevent it developing into chronic pharyngitis — a chronic inflammation of the pharynx which is often coupled with bleeding mucosa.

Another throat condition is acute laryngitis, which is an acute inflammation of the larynx. This condition is more of a respiratory infection coupled with inflammation and the effects on the voice box can be such that the patient is no longer able to speak normally and the voice is reduced to a painful rasping sound. Chronic laryngitis, i.e. long-term inflammation of the larynx, can be very difficult to overcome and thus we should be aware of the detrimental influences of smoking, drinking alcohol, abuse of the voice and unusual stress. The mucous membranes will need time to heal, just the same as with other throat conditions. Again, because of toxicity, the diet may need to be modified and the use of enemas may be considered in order to overcome such conditions much more quickly.

As all these conditions could result in hoarseness of the voice, some simple advice is to chew rowanberries. Many people think that these small berries are poisonous, but I always point out to them that if a small bird can live on them, then so can human beings — as long as they are taken in moderation.

Chronic conditions can linger as the result of an unhealthy lifestyle, and if the patient leads a stressful life, he or she should try and relax a little more. People who have a predisposition to such conditions should not forget to include watercress, sage, thyme, lemon and elder flower in the daily diet.

Extra calcium, for example, in the form of Urticalcin and Nature's Best's Calcium Citrate will expedite improvement. It is often assumed, mistakenly I must add, that throat conditions are something one has to learn to live with. Yet I am increasingly concerned about the increase in the occurrence of throat complaints, asthma and bronchitis and I believe that the blame for this must lie with environmental pollution. Unfortunately, pure air is a scarce commodity and nowhere more so than in the industrialised countries, where the extent of air pollution has become a major cause for concern. Recent reports from the London Air Pollution Monitoring Network concluded that the levels of dioxide, nitrogen-oxide, lead and other pollutants in the atmosphere are increasing. Our health and, subsequently, the quality of life is bound to deteriorate as a result and yet we can do much to protect ourselves. It is encouraging that environmentalists are aware of the increase in the present levels of pollution. It is up to each of us to protect our health and it is not fair to place that responsibility elsewhere, at the door of the government and other people who are committed to doing something about it. We can all play a part in helping to reverse this trend and in the process we will protect ourselves against these health problems.

A few years ago I became the proud owner of one of the oldest herbal practices in Britain — Napier's of

Edinburgh. Napier's was founded by a medical botanist and contained a dispensary as well as a retail outlet. My main concern was to acquire and secure for the future their wealth of herbal recipes. To my delight, many recipes dated back to the nineteenth century, when much time and effort was spent in finding cures for influenza, colds, coughs and throat conditions. Many of these recipes are still applicable today and are clearly based on common sense. I discovered a note attached to one of these old prescriptions, written by a Professor Buchanan, stating that the effect of this antidote was truly marvellous. In the books that had been compiled — full of remedies, recipes and general common sense advice — I was able to read about treatments for a quinsy throat which have long been forgotten, such as syrup of mulberries, Vick's and sal-ammoniac boiled in a little milk and used for gargling. There is an abundance of equally simple remedies, some of which I prepare sometimes for patients who have failed to find relief with some of the more modern methods. Fortunately, hundreds of these recipes have been left to us and remain available for future use. Some of these recipes may look deceptively easy, but how fortunate we are that we can enjoy the fruit of some creative genius who during the last century devoted his or her life to gaining extensive knowledge of treatments without side-effects for a large variety of diseases.

In my work I use old as well as new methods and I am thrilled to discover time and again that old and new can often successfully complement each other. Sometimes a small adjustment, achieved by osteopathic manipulation or by simple vibratory therapy, can effect positive changes. It is absolutely clear to me, from all kinds of evidence, that we cannot disassociate ourselves from the whole solar entity and remain a healthy and useful part of the earth. The earth is the womb of our solar system and has such immense beauty. Let us treasure it. Treat the body as naturally as possible, with a healthy diet and natural remedies.

On my desk I have a letter from a patient that speaks for itself! A Derbyshire lady wrote:

> "I am overjoyed to tell you that for the last month I have been completely free of asthma and all related symptoms. I have continued my treatment and am now ready for the next stage! It is a year past in June since I first visited you and if you could see me now you would know just how wonderful your cures are. I have regained my energy, my nails have strengthened and I awake each morning able to breathe easily and without effort. You will never realise how grateful I am to you. I have still got my dog, so that is not the reason for my recovery.
>
> Please advise me on the next step in the wonderful 'Freedom from Drugs' campaign."

It is wonderful to be able to live in harmony with our natural environment and deploy the gifts supplied freely in nature by our Creator.

12

Exercises and Other Therapies

DIFFERENT KINDS OF exercises, among them breathing and water exercises, are widely recommended for people who suffer from asthma and bronchitis. In this chapter I will describe some of the exercises I have successfully worked with over the years.

One form of exercise that has proved especially helpful is the Hara breathing method. In several of my books I have referred to this breathing programme, and asthma and bronchitis patients will benefit greatly if the exercises are practised regularly whilst in a state of relaxation.

Stand up straight and let your arms hang loosely beside your body, with your head dropped forward in a relaxed manner. Breathe in through the nose, into the stomach and out through the mouth. Do not interrupt this breathing pattern, but follow the natural rhythm — breathing in through the nose and out through the mouth.

During an asthma attack the patient should place his arms on a table and rest his head on his arms. Once again, breathe in deeply through the nose. If another person is present during a severe attack, it would be helpful if he or she could place an ice-cold cloth on the patient's spine between the sixth and ninth dorsal vertebra while the patient is doing this breathing exercise.

Another exercise that is always helpful is to stand erect with the feet apart and hands pressing on the abdomen. Breathe in through the nose, slowly and deeply, and breathe out slowly allowing the ribs to pull in the abdomen as much as possible.

In order to reduce the tension experienced during an attack and stimulate the circulation, stand or sit up straight with your arms folded under the chin. Do not move your shoulders, lower your chin onto the chest, turn your head to the right shoulder and raise it up again, then turn to the left and lower your chin onto the left shoulder. Return to the starting position, moving the head in as wide a circle as possible. Relax, while turning the head in a circular movement starting from the left five times, then repeating five times starting from the right.

In order to facilitate breathing through the nose when restrictions make this difficult, prepare a bowl of hot water to which a few drops of Poho oil have been added. Bend your head over the bowl and breathe deeply, in and out in a controlled rhythmic pattern. The same can be done to alleviate a sore throat.

The maxim "breathing is life" is true for everyone, but never more so than for asthmatic people. In my book *Stress and Nervous Disorders* I have mentioned an especially useful exercise from the Hara breathing method which I practise myself when things threaten to get on top of me. This breathing method specifies a number

117

of exercises that enable us to relieve depression, worry, obsession and anxieties. Once we have learned how to exercise the abdomen by rhythmic breathing, we will feel much better in ourselves. Do some breathing exercises when you wake up in the morning — and you will be set up for the day. Imagine yourself outside on a bright, crisp, even frosty day, inhaling all this oxygen in the manner described and there is no doubt that you will feel the benefits.

Clearing the bronchial tubes is essential if we are to be able to breathe through the nose. Incorrect breathing can lead to many other conditions, such as polyps or congestion, and even to deterioration of the body posture. Correct breathing will instantly reduce a bulging tummy.

Children should be taught at a young age how to develop the lungs, chest and the entire respiratory system. We can never stress this enough to the younger generation, for it must become second nature to them if they are to enjoy good health. The methods that we can use in order to achieve this are definitely not difficult, nor do they cost any money; all that is needed is a little time and consideration and any investment in this respect will certainly pay off very well in the future.

For instance, try doing a few simple exercises while standing erect. Starting with your arms hanging loosely by your sides, inhale as you raise your arms into the air, then drop your arms to the feet, at the same time bending the knees as you exhale. Stand up straight again, with relaxed shoulders and your arms hanging loose beside the body. Then raise your elbows to shoulder height as you inhale, and exhale while dropping the elbows back down beside the body.

To stimulate the diaphragm, lie flat on the floor, completely relaxed. Move your hands and feet up and down, while the muscles in the whole of the body are relaxed, then breathe in deeply through the nose and slowly out through the mouth. Repeat all these exercises several times. The routine may seem too simple to be any good, but it has a significant effect. In days gone by, tuberculosis patients staying in rest homes and sanitoria were instructed to follow exactly the same routine as part of their recovery programme.

Regular bowel movements are essential if we are to maintain a healthy constitution. Poisons from toxic waste are carried throughout the body and these must be disposed of. When the bowels do not perform their normal function regularly, it may be wise to consider an enema, although this should not be done on a regular basis as that would make the bowels lazy. In general terms, a chamomile enema will help to bring down a fever, while a sage enema has a warming and purifying action.

The well-known herbalist, Kitty Campion, has worked out a four-day cleansing fast and this programme has been used to good effect by quite a few of my patients.

Four-day cleansing fast
Fasting is done for a number of reasons, for example:

—as a way of becoming more sensitive to the body;
—for a curative effect, especially with chronic ailments;
—to lose excess weight or excess fluid;
—to clean out accumulated waste;
—to free a blockage of the energy flow in the body;
—to promote longevity;
—as a way of developing calmness, control and willpower.

A four-day cleansing fast is adequate to satisfy these concerns for most people. The method of fasting will

119

depend on the nature of the individual's usual diet and his or her constitution. For people whose diet is high in meat, the cleansing through "expansion" method is most suitable. This relies on stimulating the process of elimination, especially through the bowels. For people whose diet is predominantly vegetarian, the cleansing through "contraction" method is used. This method relies primarily on removing water from the system. In this instance a *yang* diet is one which predominates in meat and eggs while a *yin* diet is rich in raw vegetables and fruits.

Cleansing through expansion
The first three days of the fast are begun each morning with a herbal enema using a tea made with raspberry, comfrey or catnip leaves. Then, one or two 8 oz. glasses of prune juice can be taken to stimulate elimination and to help draw the toxins down into the bowels. Every two hours throughout the day, drink a glass of fresh apple juice. To stimulate the secretion of bile and elimination of toxins, take a tablespoon of olive oil with half a teaspoon of cayenne 2–4 times per day.

On the fourth day you should begin to break the fast, and after the enema and prune juice, a lunch of some lightly cooked, steamed or baked fruits or vegetables can be added and a balanced normal diet can be resumed on the fifth day.

Cleansing through contraction
Begin each day of the fast with a herbal enema using a tea made with raspberry, comfrey or catnip leaves. Eat a small bowl of brown rice three times a day, with no additional liquids. For a more effective fast, eat only one bowl of rice a day, taking a tablespoon whenever you experience strong hunger pangs, chewing the rice very

well. No other foods or drinks are to be taken during the four-day fast. However, this method of fasting may cause mild constipation and if this occurs a small bowl of stewed prunes may be taken once each day.

To break the fast, on the fifth day, take only lightly cooked fruits and vegetables, and grains. Resume a normal balanced diet high in grains on the sixth day.

This diet is excellent for eliminating excess moisture, reducing coldness of the body and restoring the ability to assimilate nutrients. It will also help to remove the sensation of excessive thirst for those who normally experience that condition.

Alternating the expansion and contraction methods

Either method of fasting may precipitate a minor healing crisis. If you do not experience a healing crisis, or achieve a significant change in your condition, it may be useful to use the opposite cleansing method. Sometimes it is necessary to alternate between expansion and contraction in order to encourage the body to excrete its toxic waste.

What is a healing crisis?

Kitty Campion has found it necessary to write about this simply because so many patients completely misunderstand what all herbalists refer to as the *law of nature*.

The healing crisis is recognised in all systems of natural healing. The Chinese refer to this as the *law of cure*. It is common, when undergoing an effective therapy, to find that the patient seems to get worse before getting better. When the body is engaged in the elimination of toxins accumulated over the years, you may experience aches, pains and symptoms of diseases, from the most recent to those of childhood. This is because the toxins are being liberated from their storage places and are now actively affecting the body with full force. This is the healing crisis.

If you experience discomfort or marked weakness during the four-day fast, or as a result of taking the herbs and recommended diet, you should strengthen your determination to go through with it. Strength and improved well-being will return when the process of elimination has been sufficiently accomplished. The cleansing fast can be repeated after one month to help complete the process.

Certain forms of hydrotherapy are often useful, especially for a cold or a fever. I heartily recommend the brush bath method, which involves gradually increasing the temperature of the water. Fill the bath with warm water (roughly body temperature); this can be best measured by immersing the elbow in the water or, if preferred, by using a thermometer. Using some soap, energetically brush the toes, the soles of the feet, the calves and steadily work up to the lumbar area of the back. When the skin has become red and glowing, after a few minutes, add some hot water to increase the temperature of the bath. This procedure can be repeated several times, until the patient begins to feel slightly uncomfortable. Then it is better to quickly get out of the bath and lie down, because perspiration may follow. This should be allowed to run its course. When the patient is really ill it may be preferable to remain in the bath while the water is cooling down. This programme can be carried out once or twice a day, as required. Sometimes it is helpful to drink a cup of hot herbal tea after such a bath, or a honey and lemon drink. For a selection of further water treatments you may wish to refer to my book *Water — Healer or Poison?* in which I discuss this subject in greater detail.

An old-fashioned, but nevertheless effective, method for bronchitis patients is to dissolve one or two dessert-spoons of kitchen salt in one litre of water at a temperature of 25°C (77°F). If possible, use something like an old nightdress, or any garment with long sleeves, and soak this thoroughly in the solution. Take care to ensure that the garment is not made of artificial fibres. Squeeze out the excess liquid and put on the garment, before lying down on a bed covered with a flannel sheet. Wrap the flannel sheet completely round your body and then cover yourself with a woollen blanket. Allow the body to perspire freely and once that has stopped completely, relax further in a nice hot bath. On a smaller scale this treatment can be done using wet stockings or socks, which can be kept on all night if wished. Put on a pair of woollen stockings or socks over the ones dipped into the salt solution and this will improve the circulation and relieve the symptoms of a cold.

Try herbal inhalation using a bowl of steaming hot water to which any of the following herbs have been added: chamomile, salvia, onions, watercress, menthol, peppermint or Poho oil. The same ingredients can also be used to prepare a herbal drink. It has been said that poor digestion can be the origin of all illness and herbal teas benefit the metabolic system as well as the digestive system. For some instructions on how to prepare herbal drinks, I will again give you some of Kitty Campion's advice.

How to make a medicinal herb tea
Herbs that have a relatively mild flavour and are to be taken internally are frequently taken as a herbal tea. When purchasing herbs for making tea, the crushed and sifted form is most useful because it is easily strained through an ordinary tea-strainer. Fresh herbs are first bruised by

rubbing between the hands or using a pestle and mortar to break down the tissue structure and release the active principles. The herbs are prepared in non-metallic containers, such as glass, earthenware or enamel pots. Stainless steel has been found to be acceptable when these are not available. Use distilled or spring water, rather than tap water, whenever possible.

The two basic methods of preparing the tea are to make an infusion or a decoction.

Infusion
If you are attempting to utilise the volatile oils in herbs such as mint or eucalyptus, or the delicate parts of the plant such as flowers and soft leaves, the herbs are steeped for 10–20 minutes in a tightly covered container with water that has just been brought to a rolling boil. This method results in what is known as an infusion. The herbs are not boiled at all, but are only steeped. A "sun tea" is made by exposing the herbs in water to the sun for a few hours in a tightly covered glass bottle.

Decoction
To extract the deeper essences from coarser leaves, stems, bark and roots, the herbs are simmered in water for about one hour. This method makes what is known as a decoction. In many cases the herbs are simmered uncovered until the volume of water has decreased by about half through evaporation. However, some of these coarser herbs contain important volatile oils (e.g. valerian, cinnamon and burdock roots) and these must be gently simmered or steeped in a covered pot.

Combining a decoction and infusion
Occasionally a formula will combine roots and bark along with soft leaves and flowers. To make a tea, a

decoction is first made with the coarser material, which is then strained and poured over the more delicate parts of the plant. This is then left to steep, tightly covered, for 10–20 minutes.

Amounts to use
Medicinal infusions and decoctions are very strong and are not like the weak teas used as a drink that most people will be familiar with. The beverage teas, such as those sold commercially in tea-bags, are made using only about one-seventh of an ounce of dried herbs per pint (two cups) of water. In contrast, the usual proportion when making a medicinal tea is one ounce of dried herbs per pint of water. The herbs will absorb some of the water, so that after making the tea, perhaps only one or one and a half cups of tea will result from using one pint of water. In most cases, this will be the correct amount for one day, since the therapy usually requires half a cup of tea to be taken three times daily. For convenience, prepare enough tea for three days of treatment all at once and keep it refrigerated in a tightly closed jar. Herbal teas will generally keep for more than three days in the refrigerator. They should be gently reheated in a covered pot before use.

If fresh herbs are used, then double the quantity given above, since much of the weight of the fresh herb is water.

As I have noted already, the standard dose of medicinal tea is half to one cup taken three times a day. Frequent small doses of two to three tablespoons (taken every half hour) will be more effective than a few larger doses when treating acute ailments.

For treatment of chronic ailments, where the herbs are to be taken over a period of several weeks, it may be more convenient to use a tincture. A tincture will also be more useful if you wish to restrict the intake of fluids. Mucilagenous herbs, such as slippery elm, comfrey root and marshmallow root, will give the tea a "slimy" quality. If this is disagreeable, the mucilagenous herbs may be taken in the form of gelatin capsules or pills along with the tea.

Illness is a disharmony and we should never stop looking for ways to harmonise the mind, body and spirit. Music and singing can be of great help in our efforts to achieve harmony. Music has the power to affect us mentally and physically and can enrich our lives. In the Far East I learned how the vibration of our lungs, voice and vocal cords can be influenced in a positive way by music. There they speak of the "healing tone". The human body can indeed be compared to a musical instrument — and perhaps it is *Life* that is playing us as though we were an instrument.

Take some time off for gentle contemplation. Close your eyes, think of a musical note and then sing that note aloud. Try and sing some melodies that derive from that note and then move around all possible melodies that are inspired by it. Every singer has a favourite key, because the resonance of that key relates to an extension of the spirit. Even singing in the shower at the top of your voice releases a message to boost your physical and mental energy. My grandmother always maintained that what happens first thing in the morning sets the tone for the remainder of that day.

A leading geologist, Dr John Waskam, has claimed that we are composed of music and light, and indeed music and light are more of a part of us than we are consciously aware. Listening to beautiful sounds or seeing a beautiful panorama is a pleasure in itself and if we are treated with music or colour, each organ and each gland will resonate a different picture and give off its own translation of the tone of life in terms of its function to make a rhythmical, musical and colourful creation. One tone, one cell, one life is a design in the realm of invisible cause and creates a panorama of music and colour. The colours in which we choose to dress ourselves are an important way of expressing our feelings and character and our search for harmony.

For healing to occur we need to look inside ourselves at our love for life, at the harmony of ourselves with our surroundings and with creation as a whole, and at the beautiful things of life on earth. It is up to us to put the right tune to it, to pitch the right tone, to sing the right tune. Once we are in harmony we can find ways to defeat illness. Often we over-estimate our efforts, because a simple melody or minor vibration can alter our lives. It was Sir Arthur Eddington who once said that: "When an electron vanishes, the universe shakes."

Glossary of Selected Herbal and Homoeopathic Remedies

Arabiaforce
Herb preparation for stimulating stomach activity, the promotion of appetite and general strengthening. Used for dyspepsia, sub-acidic gastritis, stomach cramps, nausea, change in diet and climate, and as a biliary flow stimulant.

Aloe capensis	16.2%
Nux Cola (cola nut)	16.2%
Cortex Chinae succ. (Peruvian bark)	16.2%
Fructus Auranti immat. (bitter orange)	16.2%
Rhizoma Calami (sweet myrtle)	16.2%
Gentiana lutea (yellow gentian)	10.0%
Gummi Myrrhae (myrrh)	4.5%
Olibanum elect. (frankincense)	4.5%

Asthma drops
A fresh herb preparation for bronchial asthma and congestion of the lungs. Anti-spasmodic.

Ephedra vulg.	20%
Urag. ipecacuanha 6x	15%
Crataegus oxyacantha (hawthorn berry)	10%
Carduus benedictus (blessed thistle)	5%

Pimpinella saxifraga (burnet saxifrage)	5.0%
Thymus vulg. (thyme)	5.0%
Grindelia robusta (gum plant)	1.0%
Spongia tosta 1x	0.2%
Kalium iodatum 1x	0.1%

Bronchosan
Anti spasmodic and relaxant – particularly in bronchial spasm, stimulates secretions of bronchial mucosa.

Convascillan (*Convallaria* combination)
A fresh herb preparation for nervous heart problems, senile heart, heart stress, myocardial weakness following infections, palpitations and feelings of anxiety.

Convallaria majalis (lily of the valley)	94.5%
Convallaria juice	5.0%
Scilla maritima	0.5%

Drosinula cough syrup
A pure herb syrup, soothing for inflammations of the respiratory tract. Used for whooping cough, coughs due to colds, irritation due to coughing, and stubborn, severe and deep cough. Also useful as an aid to treating bronchial asthma.

Succus Piceae abietis	
(juice of fresh double spruce)	18.93%
Drosera rotundifolia (sundew)	2.10%
Inula helenium (elecampane)	2.10%
Hedera helix (ivy)	0.55%
Urag. ipecacuanha (ipecac)	0.55%
Coccus cacti	0.05%

In a base of pear concentrate, honey and unrefined sugar.

Echinaforce
A fresh herb preparation for non-specific stimulant therapy. Echinaforce brings about an increase in the body's own resistance in the case of inflammations and infections, or susceptibility to colds and other infections. A preventative remedy for colds and cold-related infections. Used for the internal treatment of certain dermatological problems or septic processes (carbuncles, abscesses, etc.). The processes of inflammation are reduced and faster healing is promoted.

Echinacea purpurea herba	95%
Echinacea purpurea radix	5%

Galeopsis ochroleuca (hemp nettle)
A fresh herb preparation with an expectorant effect in cases of bronchial cough, problems with the respiratory tract and asthma.

Goldengrass tea (kidney tea)
Stimulates the kidney function, urinary discharge and acts as a mild disinfectant. May be used in conjunction with Nephrosolid.

Solidago virgaurea (goldenrod)	40%
Betula alba (white birch)	30%
Polygonum aviculare (knotgrass)	15%
Equisetum arvense (horsetail)	10%
Viola tricolor (wild pansy)	5%

Harpagophytum
Used to treat metabolic dysfunctions; rheumatism and arthritis; liver and gallbladder dysfunctions; kidney and bladder problems; allergies; and symptoms of advanced age.

Harpagophytum procumbens (devil's claw)

Herbamare (Herbal seasoning salt)

Herbamare is made according to the original formula of the famous Swiss naturopath Dr A. Vogel and is prepared with fresh, organically grown herbs. The fresh herbs are combined with natural sea salt and allowed to "steep" for 6–8 weeks before the moisture is removed by a special vacuum process at a low temperature. This slow, careful process allows all the good qualities, the aroma and taste to be absorbed by the sea salt. Use Herbamare at the table, in cooking or any time you want the taste and aroma of fresh herbs.

Sea salt	Celery leaves
Leeks	Celery root
Watercress	Garden cress
Onions	Chives
Parsley	Lovage
Basil	Marjoram
Rosemary	Thyme
Kelp	

Immunoforce (Formula IMN)

Stimulates and builds up the body's defence mechanism, especially when taken regularly over an extended period. Used to treat fevers and feverish illnesses. Acts as an antibacterial and antiviral medicine.

Echinacea angustifolia 3x
Eupatorium perfoliatum 2x
Aconitum napellus 4x
Thuja occidentalis 12x
Baptisia tinctoria 3x
Sambucus nigra 3x

Imperatoria

A fresh herb preparation for gastric and intestinal disorders. A diuretic. Used to treat gout, rheumatism, arthritis, asthma, bronchial catarrh and inflammation of the throat.

Imperatoria ostruthium
Peucdanum ostruthium (masterwort)

Influaforce
A homoeopathic remedy for influenza (flu) and related illnesses: acute colds, fever, neuralgia, laryngitis.

Avena sativa
Solidago virgaurea
Baptisia
Lachesis
Echinacea
Bryonia alba
Aconitum napellus

Kelpasan
Pure sea algae from the Pacific Ocean with all the trace elements. A natural supplement for iodine deficiency; a prophylaxis for goitre. Stimulates the cell metabolism of the endocrine glands. Increases mental and physical capacity.

Algae marinae sicc.
Excip. pro compr.

Lachesis
Recommended for the following conditions:
—infections, tonsillitis, inflammation of the lining membrane of the heart (endocarditis), peritonitis;
—septic processes, boils (carbuncles), blood poisoning, cellulitis;
—problems during the menopause;
—abnormally dilated veins (varicose), arteries or lymph vessels, phlebitis;
—migraine headaches;
—angina (stenocardial) attacks.

Marum verum (Cat thyme)
Used to treat insomnia, neuralgia, difficulty in swallowing, inflammation of the gums, a runny nose and pharyngitis.

133

Molkosan

Molkosan is produced from fresh Alpine whey by a natural fermentation process. It contains all the important minerals found in fresh whey, such as magnesium, potassium and calcium in concentrated forms. Molkosan is rich in natural dextrorotatory L (+) lactic acid, which in health-oriented nutrition as well as natural healing methods has a special significance.

Use Molkosan as a substitute for vinegar in all salad dressings or add one tablespoon to a glass of mineral water for a refreshing cold drink or add to vegetable juices for a little extra zip.

Recommended uses — *internally:*
—weight control — improves the metabolism;
—encourages and maintains healthy intestinal flora;
—indigestion;
—stimulates secretion of gastric acid;
—sore throats (gargle with 1 part Molkosan and 2 parts water for soothing relief and faster recovery);
—mouth disinfectant (wash out using same dilution as for gargling).

Recommended uses — *externally:*
—minor cuts and abrasions;
—athlete's foot and other skin and nail mycosis (diluted 1 to 1 with water);
—eczema, skin impurities (use externally and internally).

Nephrosolid (Kidney drops)

A fresh herb preparation to stimulate the kidney function, treat kidney and bladder problems and increase urinary discharge. Used as a support in the treatment of kidney infection. Recommended for cystitis as a result of colds. Encourages the natural urge to urinate.

Solidago virgaurea (goldenrod)	50%
Potentilla anserina (silverweed)	14%
Betula alba (birch)	13%
Ononis spinosa (restharrow)	5%
Viola tricolor (wild pansy)	5%
Polygonum aviculare (knotweed)	5%
Equisetum arvense (horsetail)	4%
Juniperus communis (juniper)	4%

Petaforce
For pain that is spasmodic or severe, in migraine headaches, menstrual pain and general pain.

Petasan syrup
Used to treat chronic complaints of respiratory tract. Protects the mucous membranes and the bronchial area. Strengthens resistance naturally. Recommended for asthmatic difficulties.

Succus Piceae abietis	
(juice of fresh double spruce)	18.6%
Petasites off. (butterbur)	7.0%

In a base of pear concentrate, honey and unrefined sugar.

Plantaforce
Plantaforce is a vegetable concentrate that is unsurpassed in quality or taste. Use it to make a delicious vegetable broth or as a seasoning for soups, stews, gravies, sauces, etc. It is especially good mixed in rice (while cooking) or noodles (after cooking). For broth, use half a teaspoon to 6–8 oz. of water; for seasoning, use to taste.

135

Hydrolised vegetable protein	Sea salt
Peanut oil	Tomato pulp
Cultured yeast extract	Green pepper pulp
Watercress	Parsley
Basil	Thyme
Celery	Leeks
Onions	Chives
Marjoram	Rosemary
Kelp	

Poho oil
A potent, effective combination of essential oils for use in alleviating the symptoms of colds and sore throats, as well as coughs and hoarseness. Also used to disinfect the mouth and throat cavity.

Essential oils:	
Menthae piperita (peppermint)	50%
Eucalyptus	30%
Juniper	14%
Carum carvi (caraway)	4%
Foeniculum vulgare (fennel)	2%

Poho ointment
For application in the case of colds, runny nose, frontal sinusitis, as well as for minor injuries.

Ol. Hyperici (St John's wort oil)	21.0%
Ol. Menthea japon. (peppermint oil)	9.5%
Aqua Hamamelidis (witch hazel water)	8.0%
Menthae piperita (peppermint)	7.5%
Calendula off.	2.0%
Ol. Citri (citrus oil)	2.0%
Extr. Hamamelidis fluid (witch hazel extract)	0.5%
Balsamum peruvianum (balsam of Peru)	0.5%

Pollinosan (hay fever formula)
Used for hay fever and similar allergies accompanied by sneezing, itching in the throat and eyes, asthma, dry hacking cough and burning, itching, runny eyes.

> *Larrea mexicana* 2x
> *Okoubaka aubrevillei* 2x
> *Cardiospermum* 2x
> *Galphimia glauca* 3x
> *Luffa perculata* 3x
> *Aralia racemosa* 2x

Rasayana no. 1
Cleanses and purifies the blood, and affects the glandular function in the intestines. As a laxative it stimulates elimination without becoming habit-forming. Also acts as a mild diuretic.

Cort. Frangulae (buckthorn bark)	17.5 mg
Extr. Aloe (aloe)	17.5 mg
Fol. Sennae (senna leaves)	17.5 mg
Fol. Uvae ursi	17.5 mg
Fruct. Foeniculi (fennel)	17.5 mg
Herba Cardui benedicti (blessed thistle)	17.5 mg
Herba Cichorii (chicory)	17.5 mg
Herba Fumariae (fumitory)	17.5 mg
Rad. Ebuli (dwarf elder)	17.5 mg
Rad. Helenii (elecampane)	17.5 mg
Rad. Ononidis (restharrow)	17.5 mg
Rhiz. Asari (wild ginger)	17.5 mg

Rasayana no. 2
Affects the liver and gallbladder. Increases the secretion of bile in cases of liver dysfunction.

Rhiz. Curcumae (Indian saffron)	95.0 mg
Extr. Aloe (aloe)	17.5 mg

Herba Centauri (centaury)	17.5 mg
Herba Hyperici (St John's wort)	17.5 mg
Rad. Taraxaci (dandelion)	17.5 mg
Rhiz. Graminis (quickgrass)	17.5 mg
Rad. Sarsaparillae (sarsaparilla)	17.5 mg
Cort. Berberidis (barberry bark)	1.75 mg
Lycopodium clavatum (club moss)	1.75 mg

Santasapina cough syrup

A cough syrup prepared from the extract of fresh pine shoots and honey. Fortifies and strengthens the respiratory tract, especially during periods of increased danger of contagion and during cold weather. Used to treat coughs, hoarseness and inflammation of the mucous membranes. The defences of the body are fortified by natural means. Honey promotes the loosening of tough mucus when coughing.

Succus Pyri comm. conc.	
(juice of fresh double spruce)	20%
Mel (honey)	24%

In a base of pear concentrate, honey and unrefined sugar.

Symphytum officinalis

Symphytum officinalis is a fresh herbal preparation that is used for the soothing effect that it gives to cases of inflammation, bruising, sprains, strains, breaks in bones, as well as phlebitis. It is also used as a blood astringent, and it helps to promote the healing of wounds of varying severity.

Urticalcin
A homoeopathic calcium and silicic acid preparation for use where a lack of calcium is indicated. Helps to build up the bones. Recommended during pregnancy and while nursing, as well as for brittle nails and loss of hair. Also has preventative effect against an excessive accumulation of acid in the body.

> *Urtica dioica* 1x
> *Silicea* 6x
> *Calcarea carbonica* 4x
> *Calcarea phosphorica* 6x
> *Natrium phosphorica* 6x
> *Excip. pro compr.*

Usneasan
A fresh herb extract for colds and cold-related illnesses, such as coughs and inflammation of the mucous membranes of the throat and bronchial tubes. Protects the mucous membranes of the respiratory tract. Activates the body's defence mechanism against colds and cold-related illnesses.

Lichen islandicus (Iceland moss)	40%
Usnea barbata (beard moss)	30%
Plantago lanceolata (lanceleaf plantain)	15%
Petasites off. (butterbur)	5%
Pinus silvestris (Scotch pine)	5%
Larix decidua (larch)	5%

Usneasan cough lozenges
Made with fresh herb extracts, and used for coughs and hoarseness. Have an antibacterial effect against germs in the mouth and throat, as well as combating any susceptibility to throat infections.

GLOSSARY

Rhiz. Iridis (blue flag)	3.03 mg
Lichen islandicus (Iceland moss)	2.80 mg
Usnea barbata (beard moss)	1.10 mg
Plantago lanceolata (lanceleaf plantain)	1.04 mg
Extr. Petasitidis (butterbur)	0.33 mg
Larix decidua (larch)	0.33 mg
Pinus silvestris (Scotch pine)	0.33 mg

Bibliography

Harry Benjamin, *Everybody's Guide To Nature Cure,* Thorsons Publishing Group, Wellingborough, Northants, United Kingdom.

Dr Elizabeth Evans, *Diet and Nutrition,* Octopus Books Limited, London, United Kingdom.

Barbara Griggs, *The Home Herbal,* Jill Norman and Hobhouse, London, United Kingdom.

Dorothy Hall, *The Natural Health Book,* Thomas Nelson, Melbourne, Australia.

Dr Rudolf Kinsky, *Ontpsan U,* De Driehoek, Amsterdam, the Netherlands.

Martin Koje, *Zelfgenezing van Nerveusiteit,* Servire, the Hague, the Netherlands.

D. Napier and Sons, *Herbs, Roots and Barks,* Ernest Kohler and Son, Edinburgh, United Kingdom.

Dr Alfred Vogel, *The Nature Doctor: A Manual of Traditional Medicine,* Mainstream Publishing Co. Ltd, 7 Albany Street, Edinburgh EH1 3UG, United Kingdom.

Dr Alfred Vogel, *De Natuur wijst de weg,* A. Vogel Verlag, Teufen, Switzerland.

The Merck Manual (14th Edition), Sharpe and Dohme Ltd, Hoddesdon, Herts, United Kingdom.

Useful Addresses

Bioforce (UK) Ltd
Olympic Business Park
Drybridge Road
Dundonald
Ayrshire KA2 9BE

Nature's Best Health Products Ltd
Freepost
PO Box 1
Tunbridge Wells
TN2 3EQ
United Kingdom

Obbekjaer's Peppermint
J. W. Bennett & Son
Wheelton
Chorley
Lancs
United Kingdom